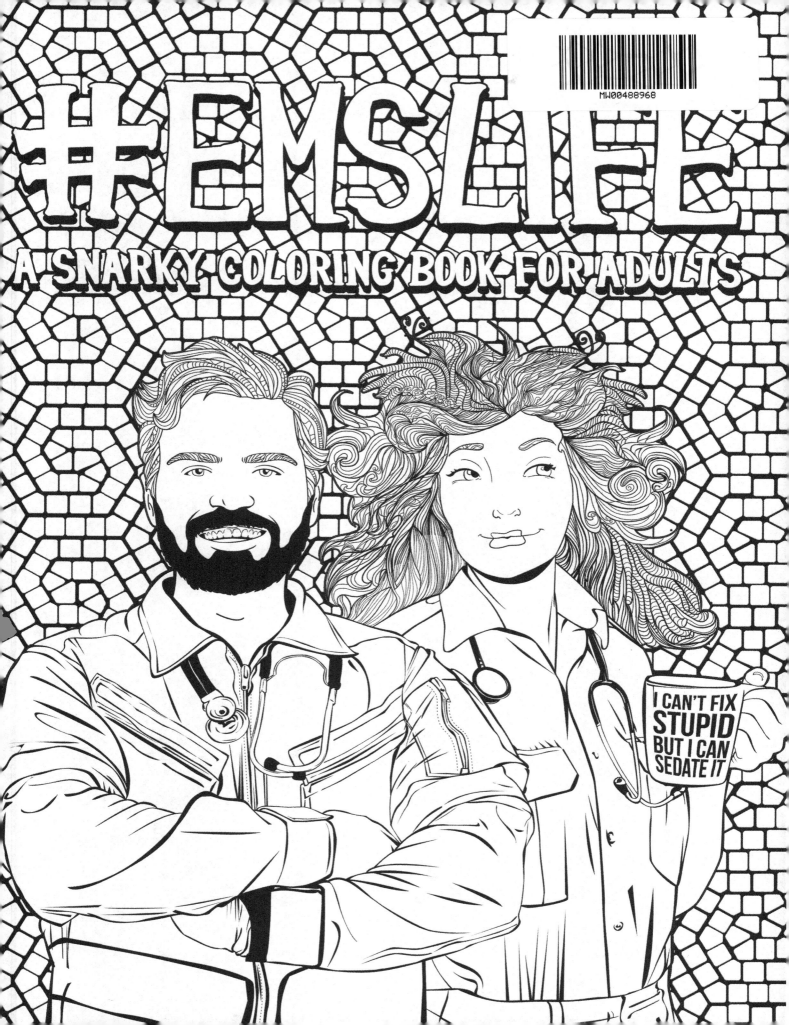

Want free goodies?
Email us at freebies@pbleu.com

@papeteriebleu

Papeterie Bleu

Shop our other books at
www.pbleu.com

Wholesale distribution through Ingram Content Group
www.ingramcontent.com/publishers/distribution/wholesale

For questions and customer service, email us at
support@pbleu.com

© Papeterie Bleu. All rights reserved. No part of this publication may be reproduced, distributed, or transmitted, in any form or by any means, including photocopying, recording, or other electronic or mechanical methods, without prior written permission of the publisher, except in the case of brief quotations embodied in critical reviews and certain other noncommercial uses permitted by copyright law.

FREE PDF DOWNLOAD
OF THIS BOOK

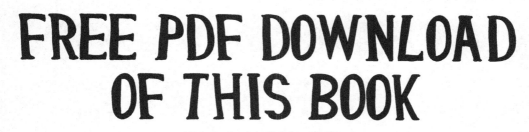

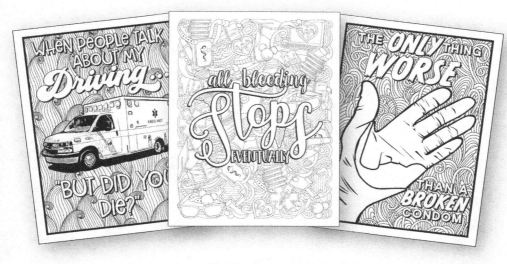

www.pbleu.com/ems

YOUR DOWNLOAD CODE: EMS373

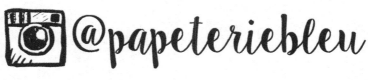 @papeteriebleu

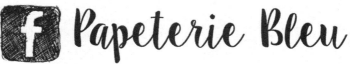 Papeterie Bleu

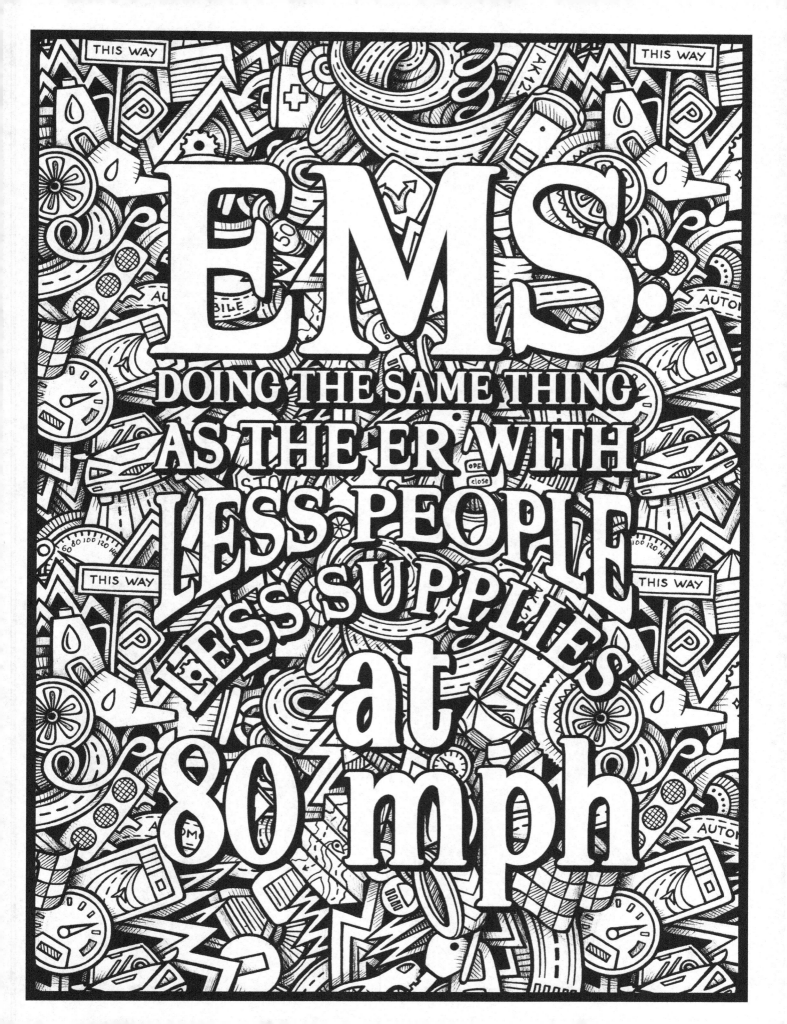

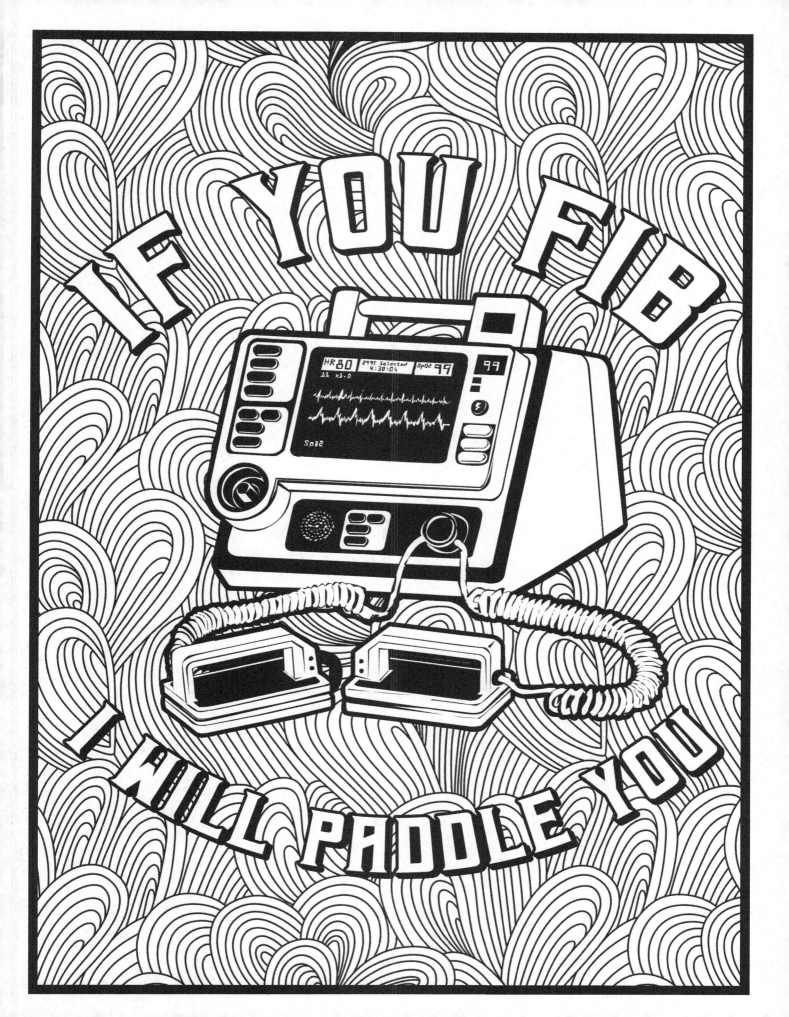

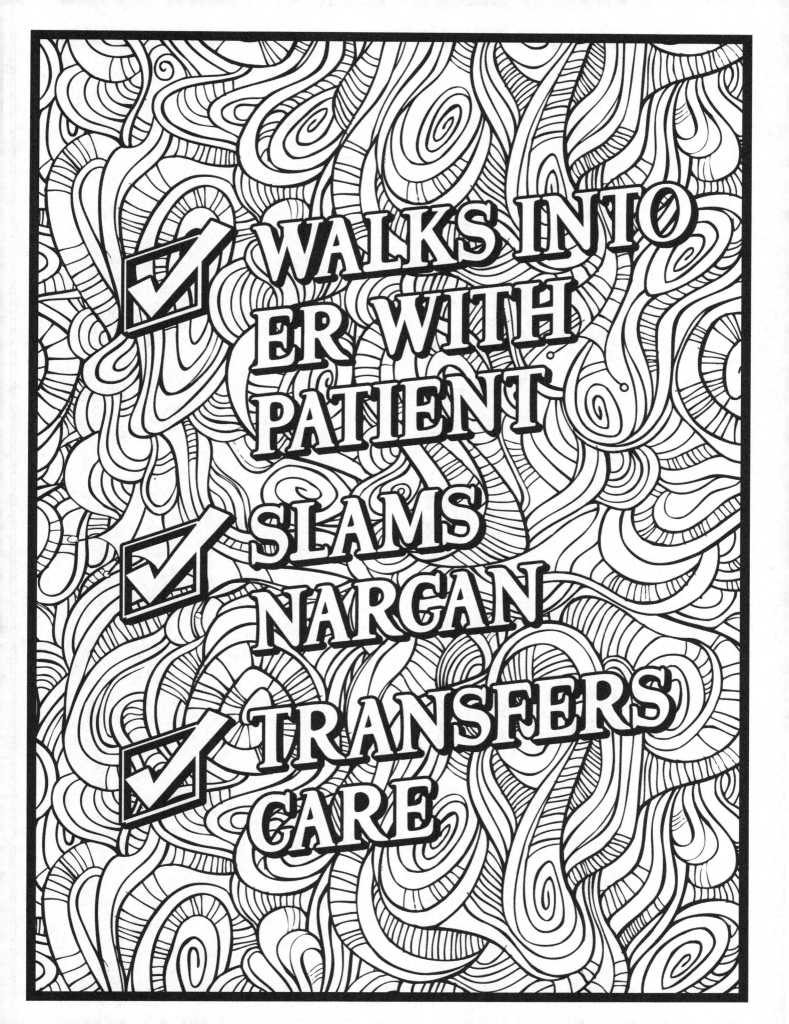

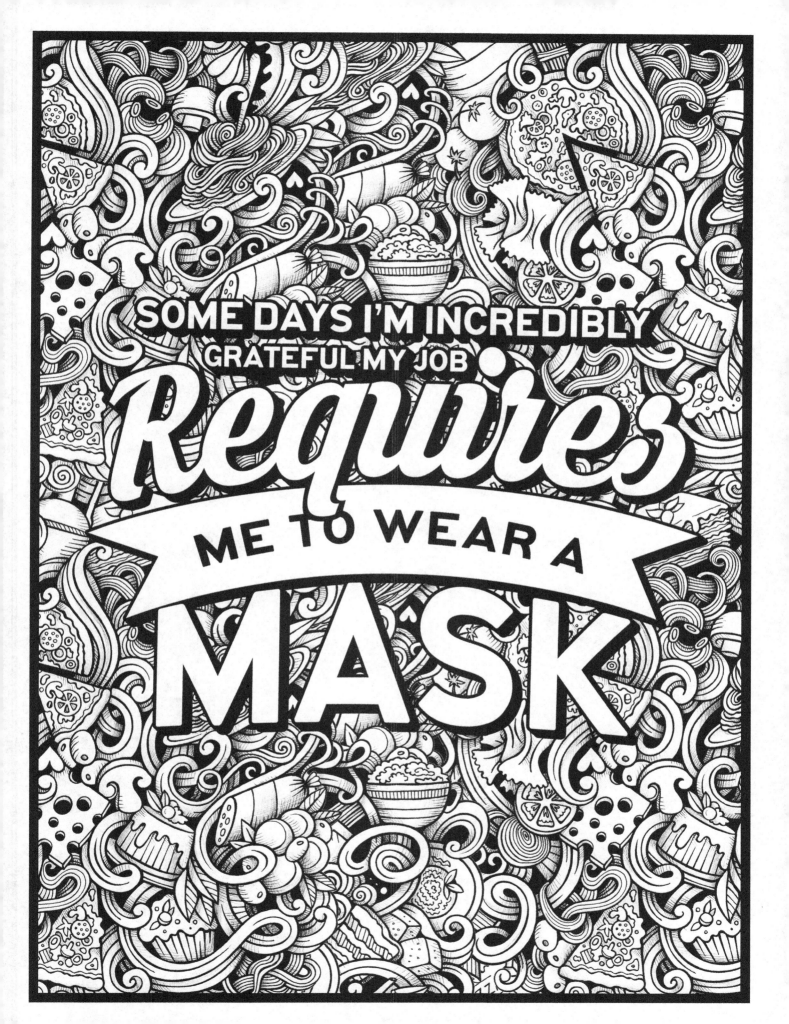

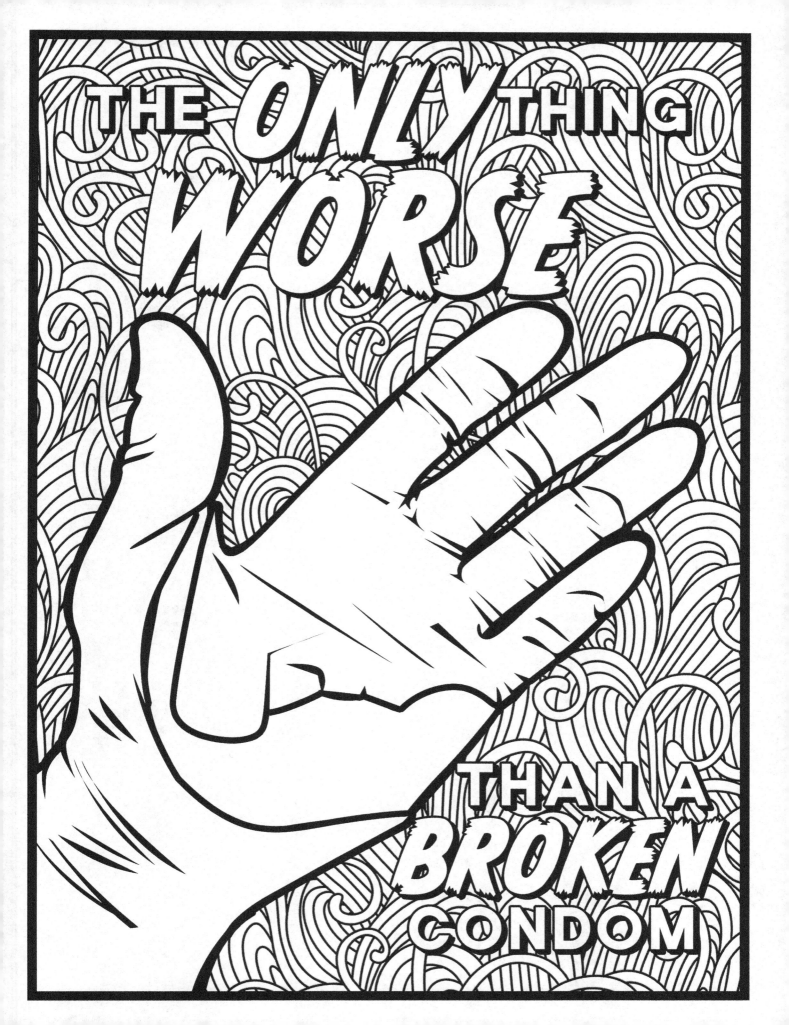

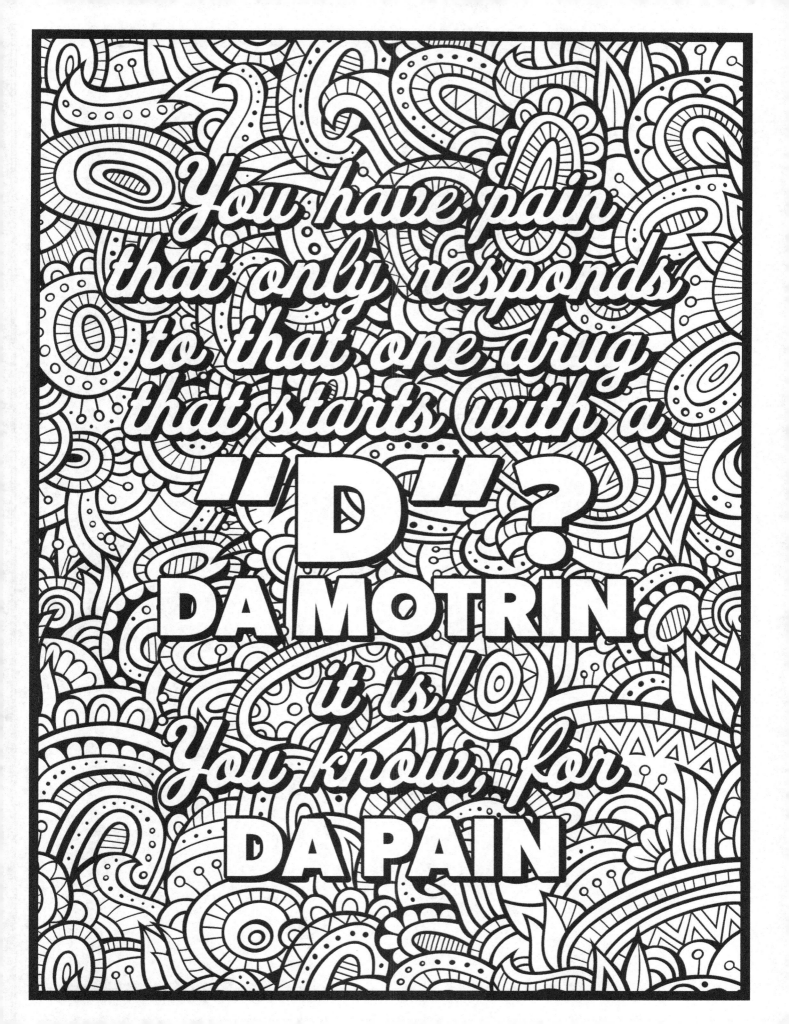

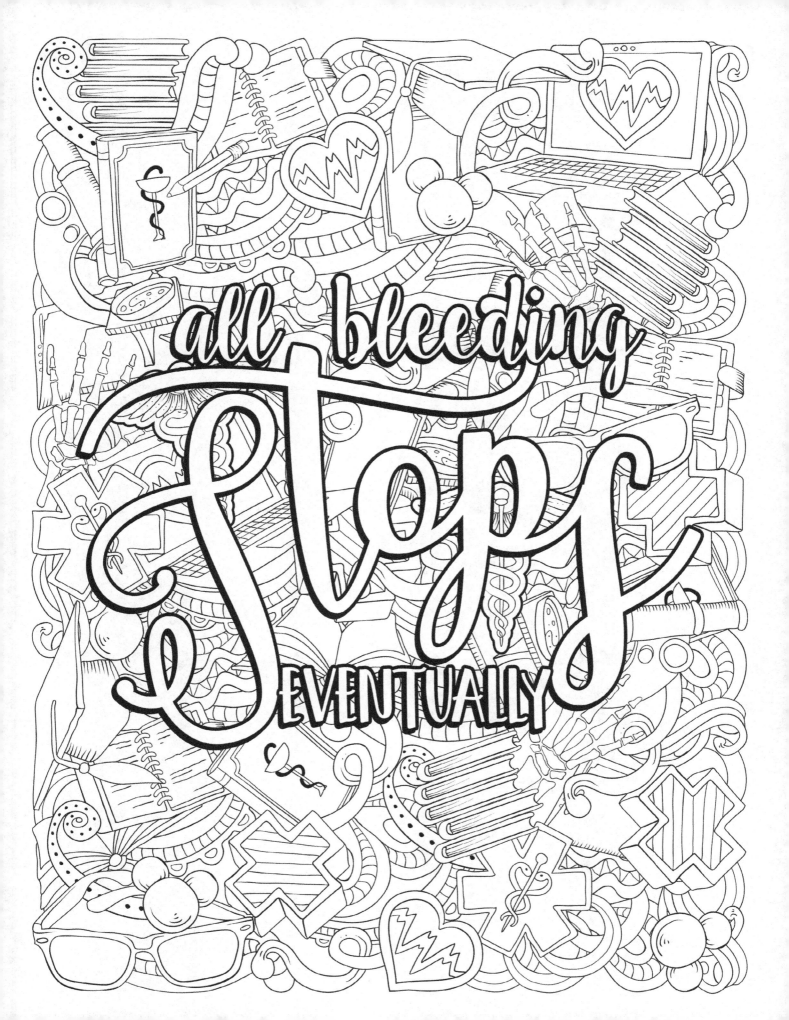

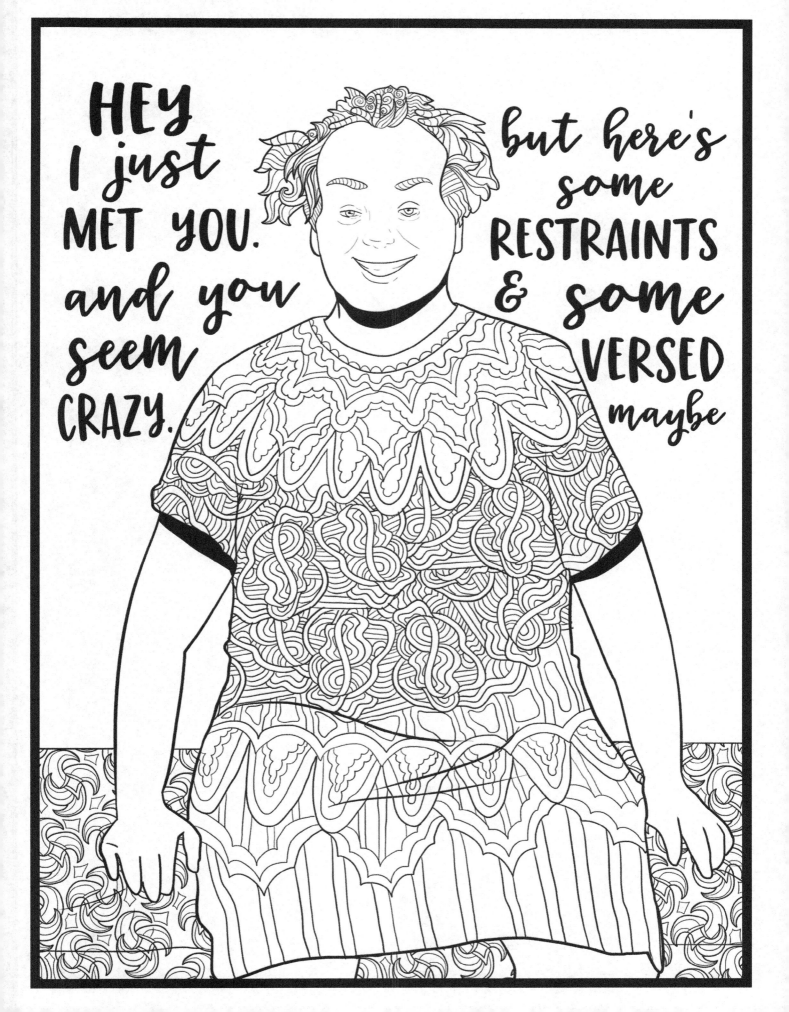

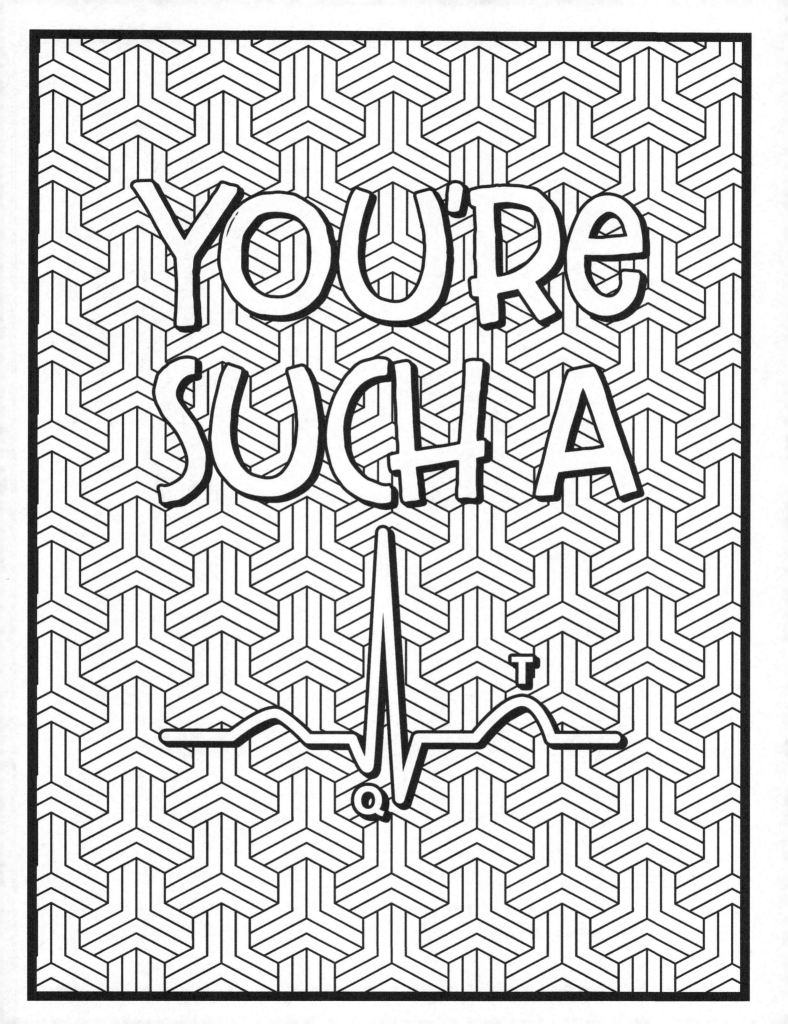

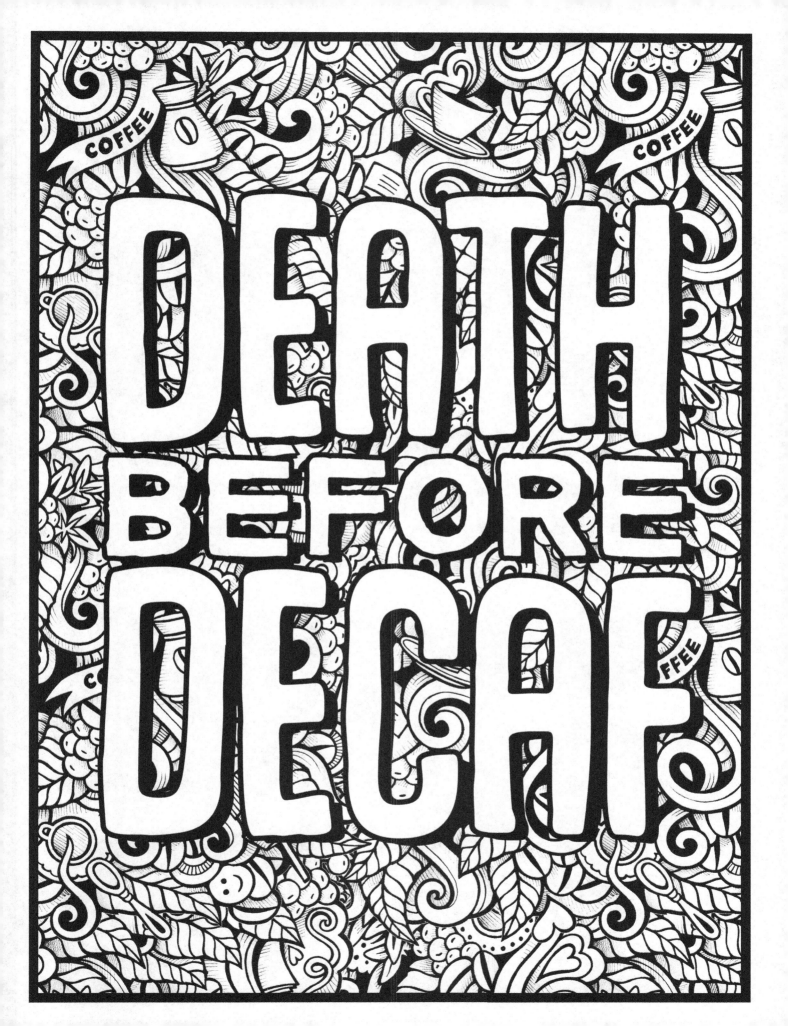

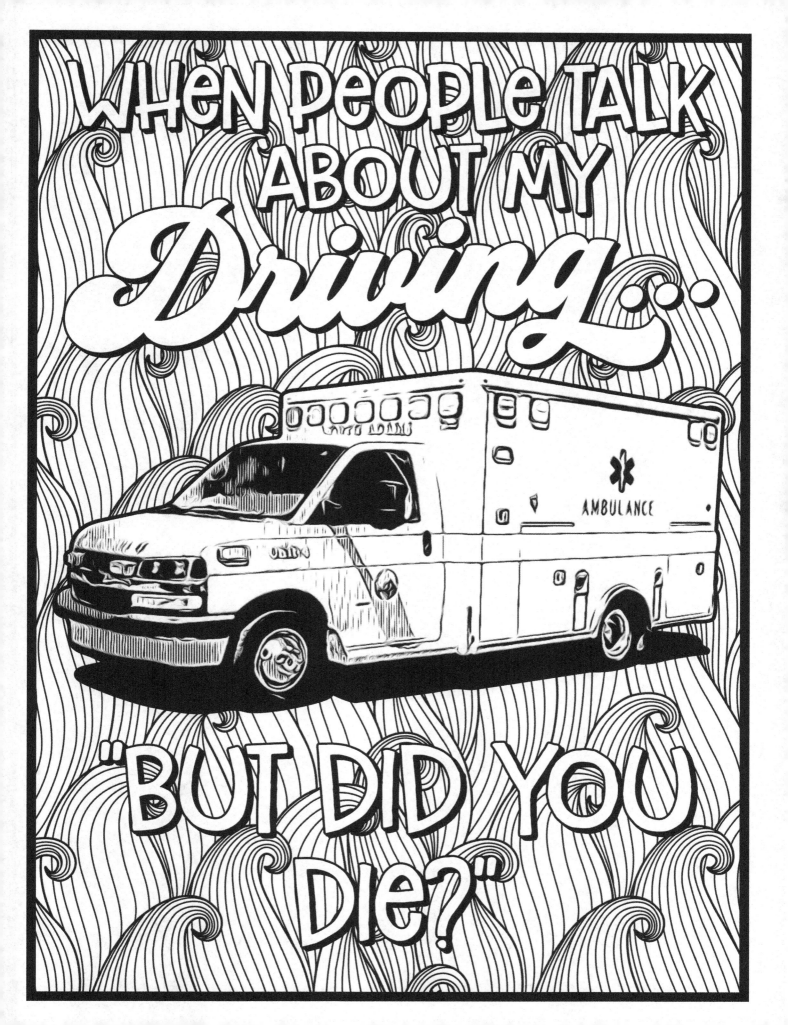

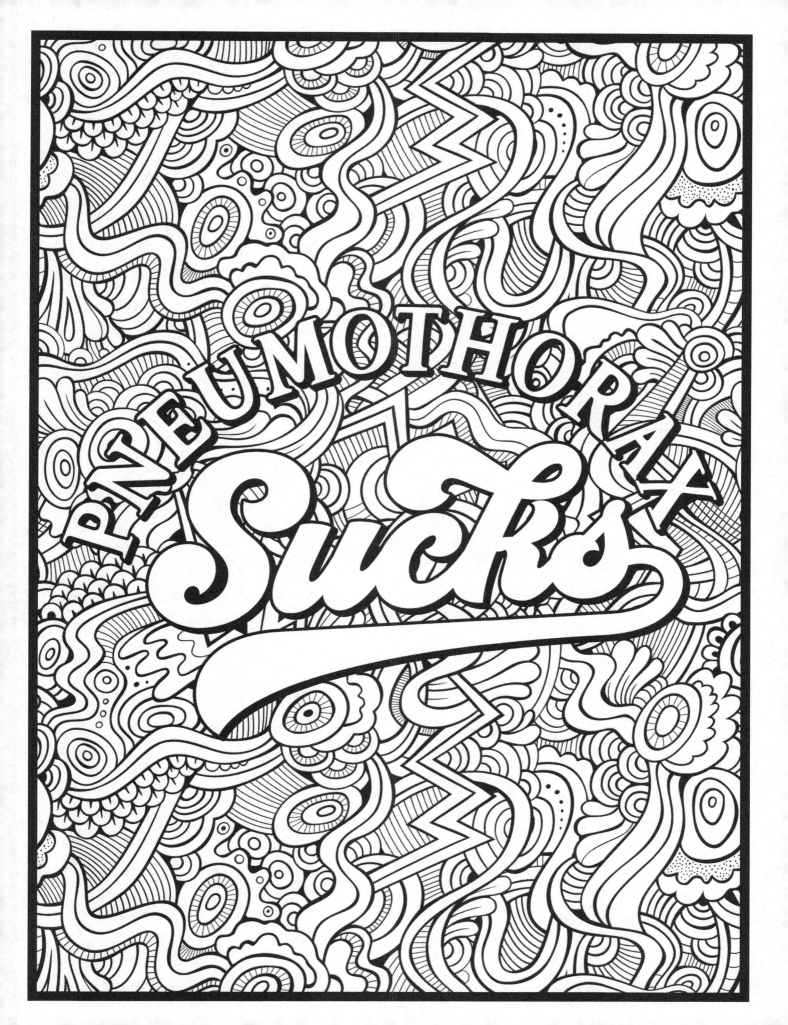

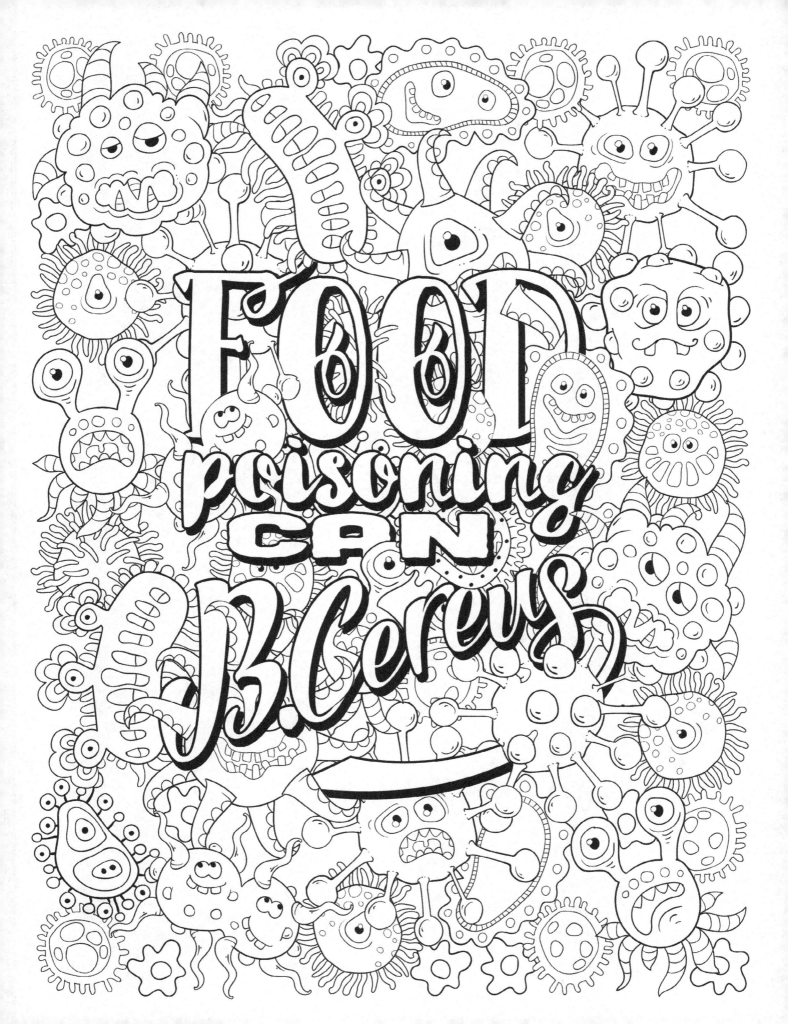

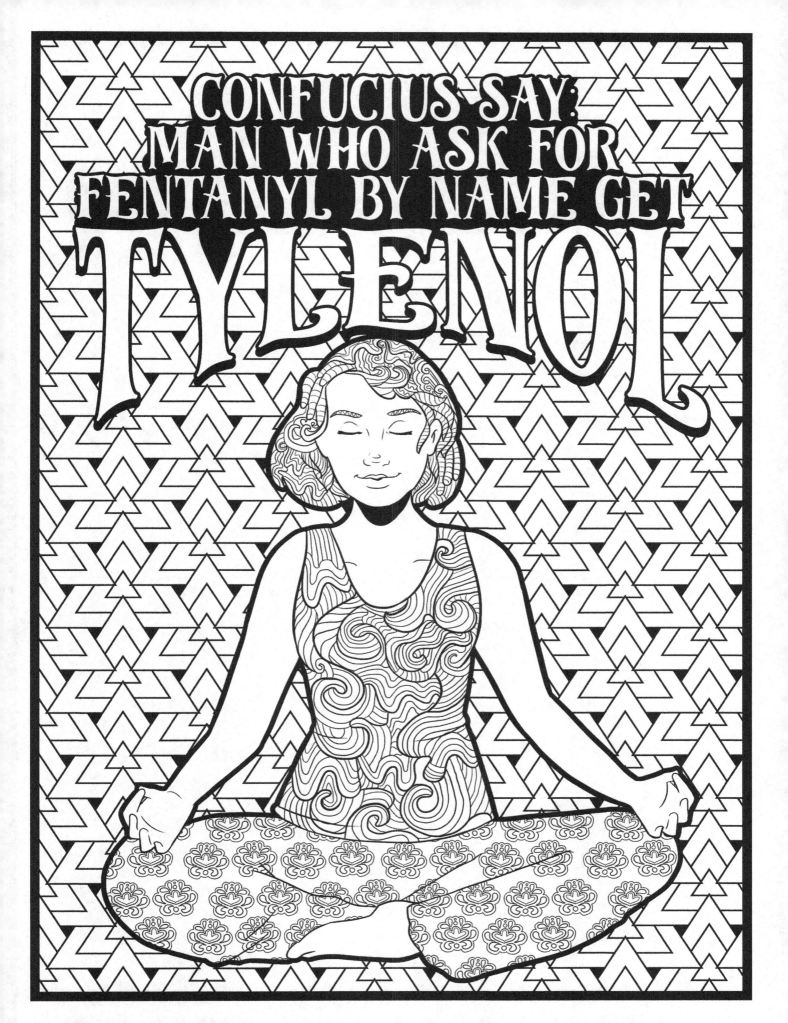

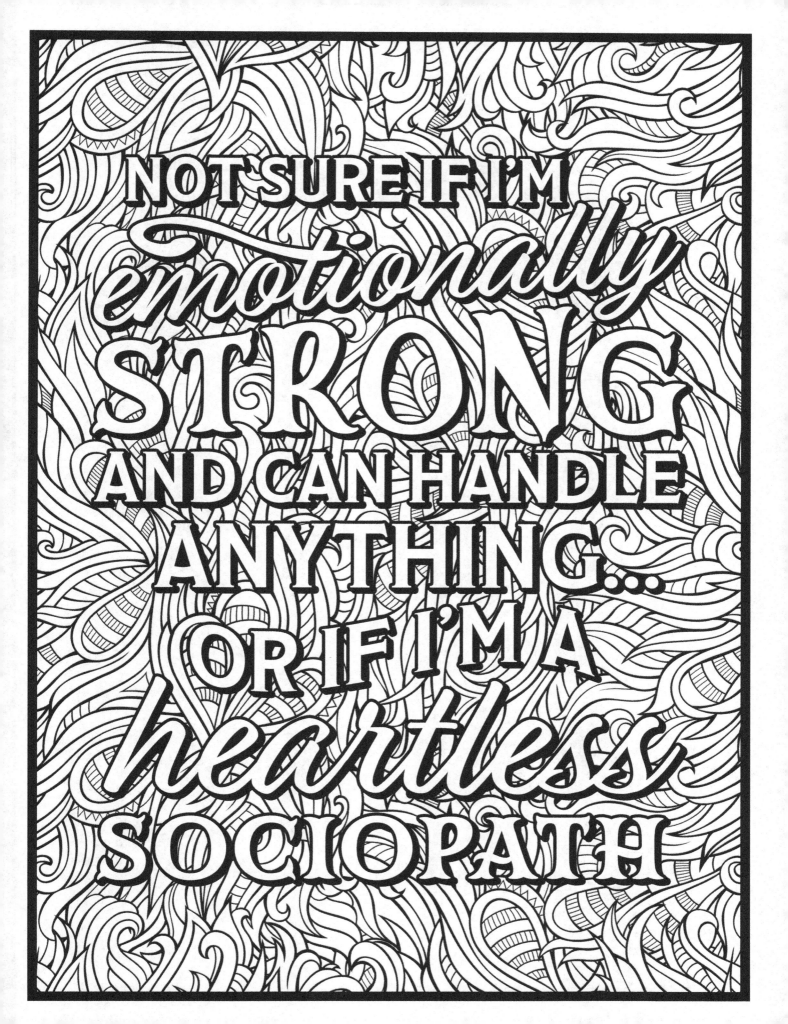

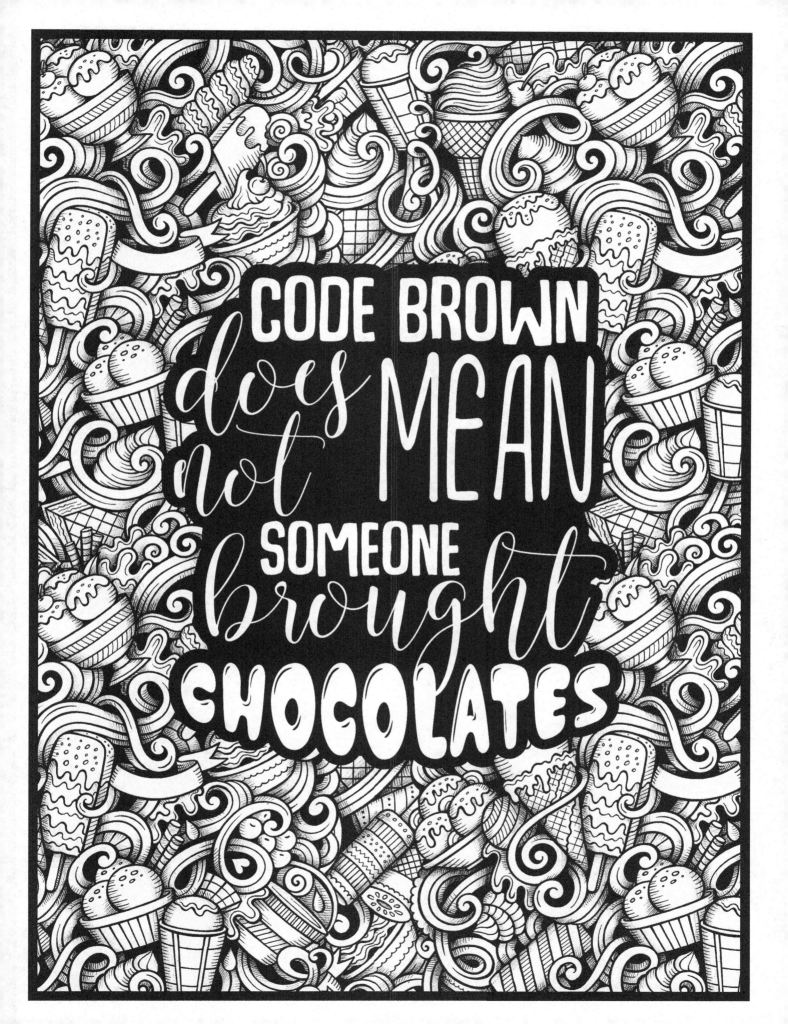

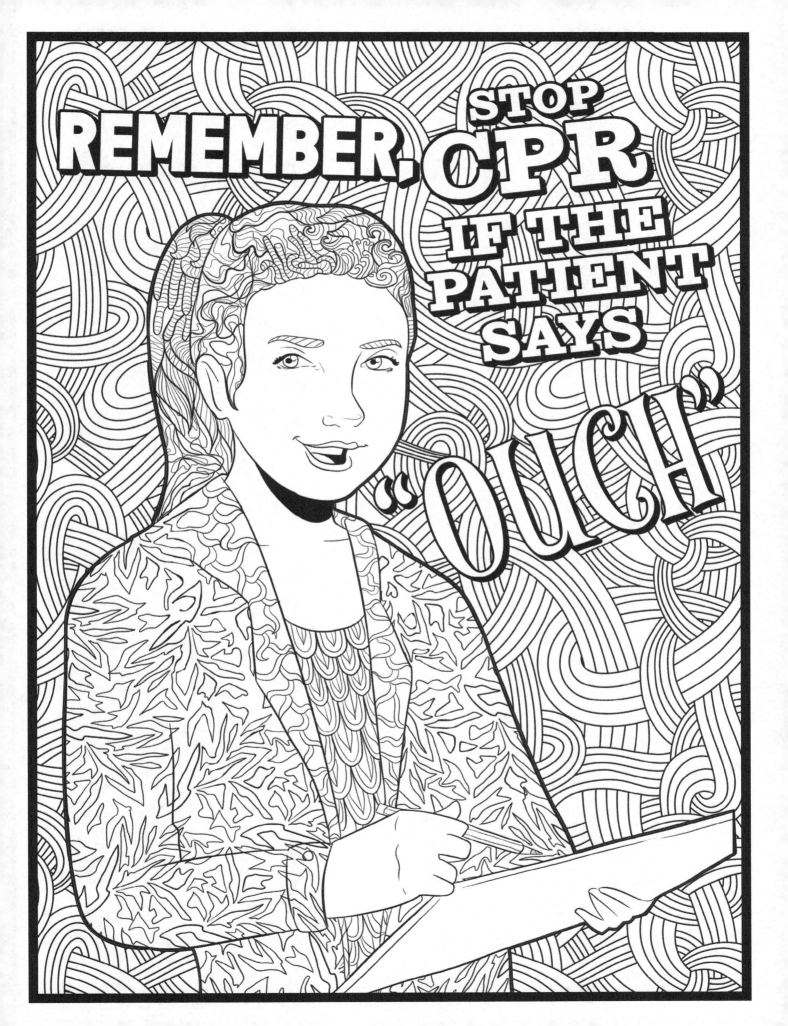

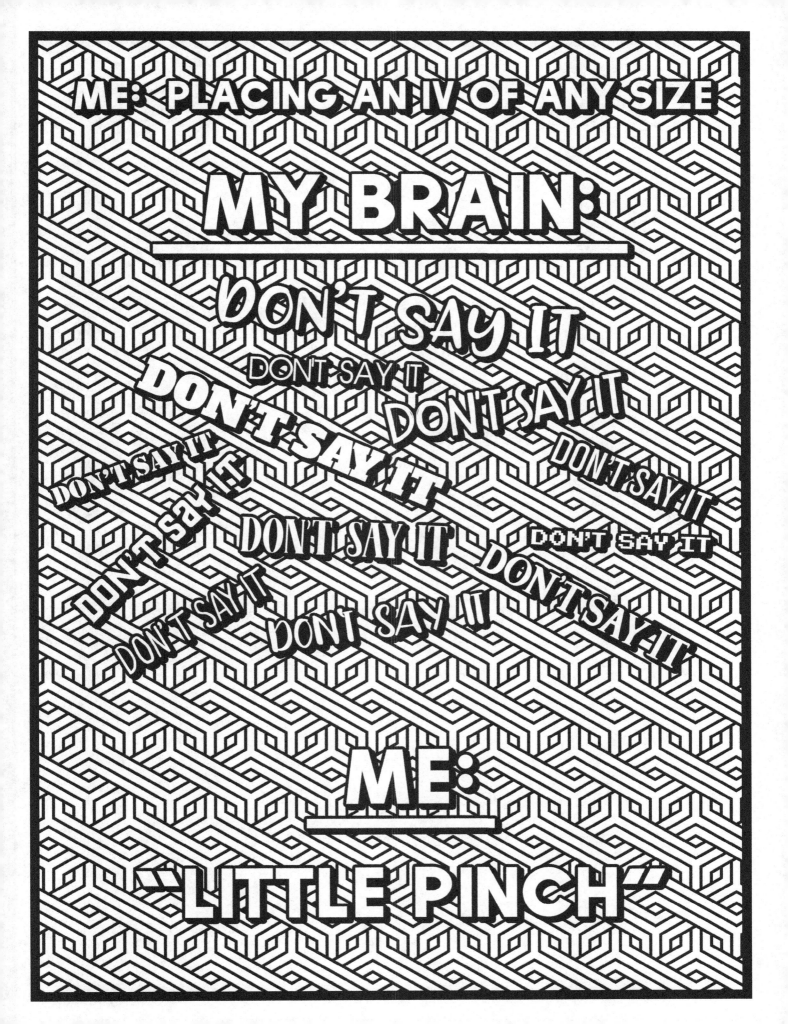

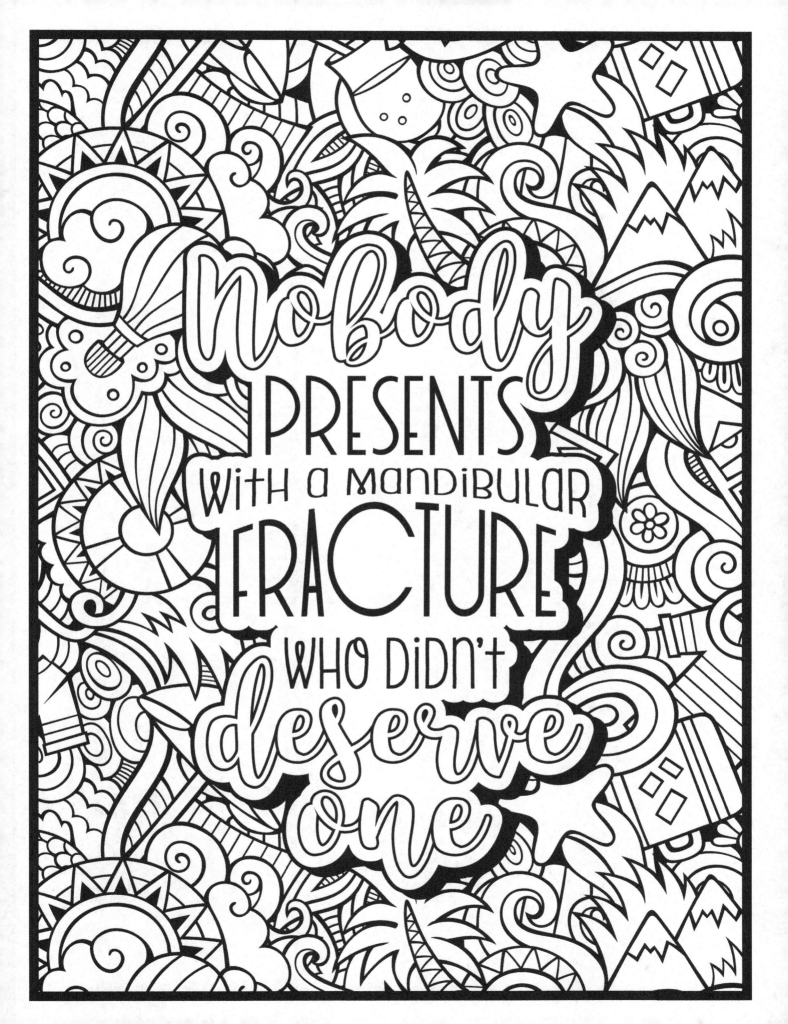

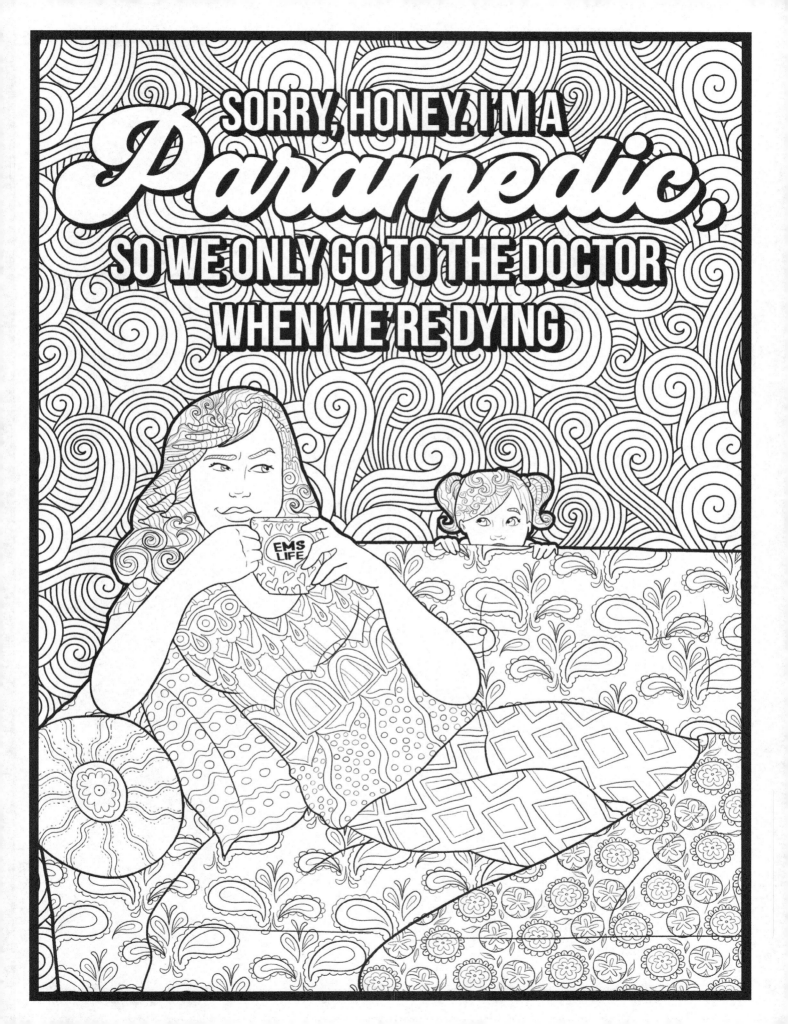

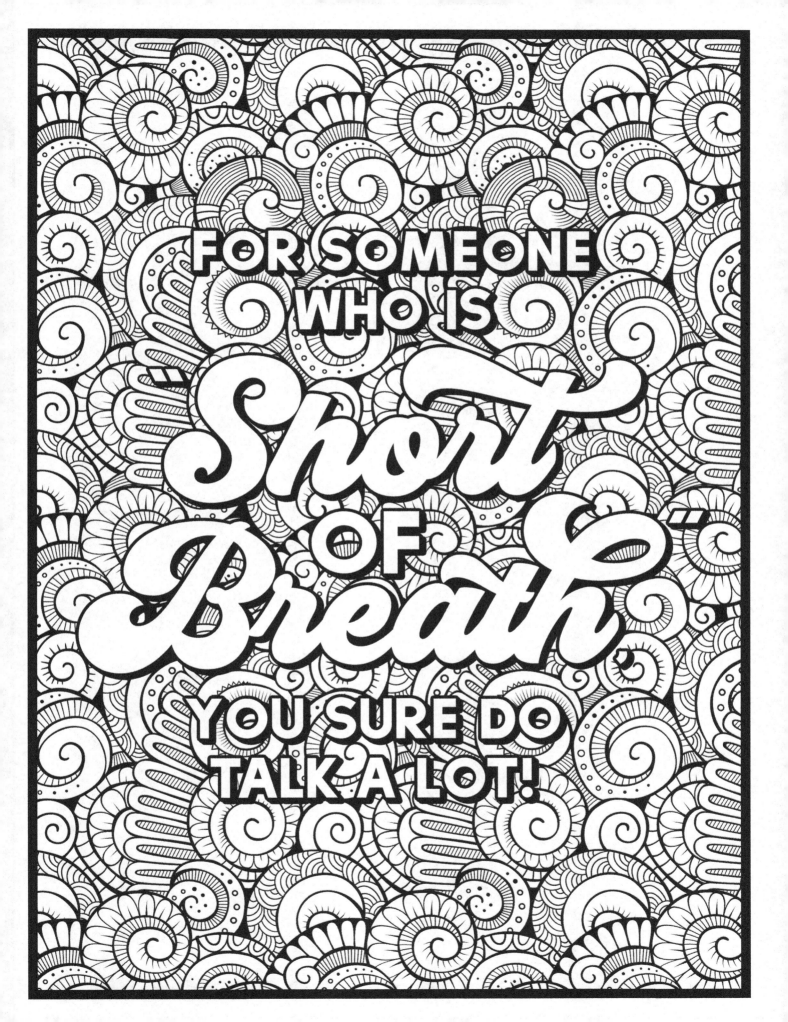

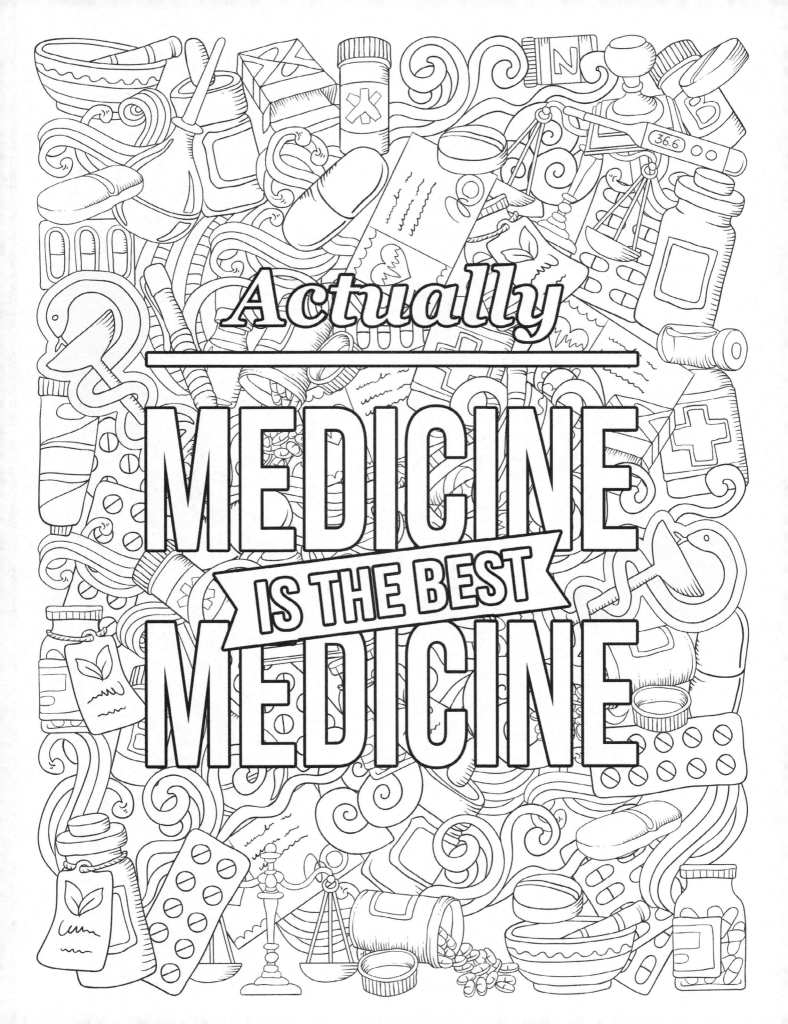

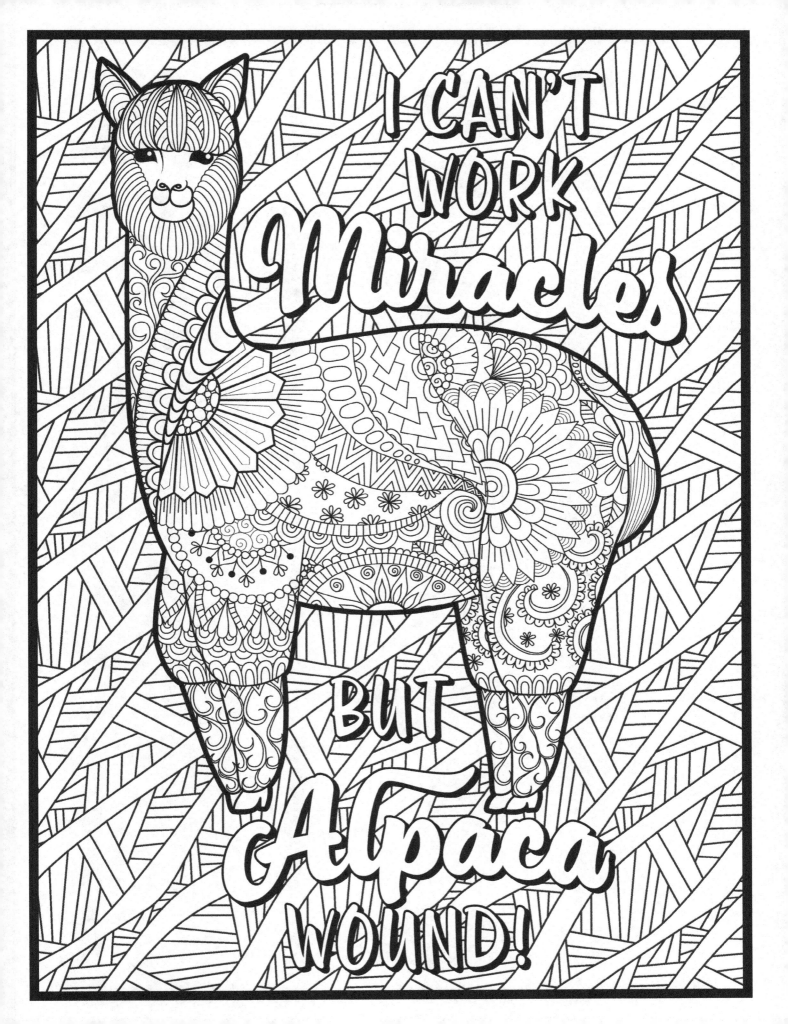

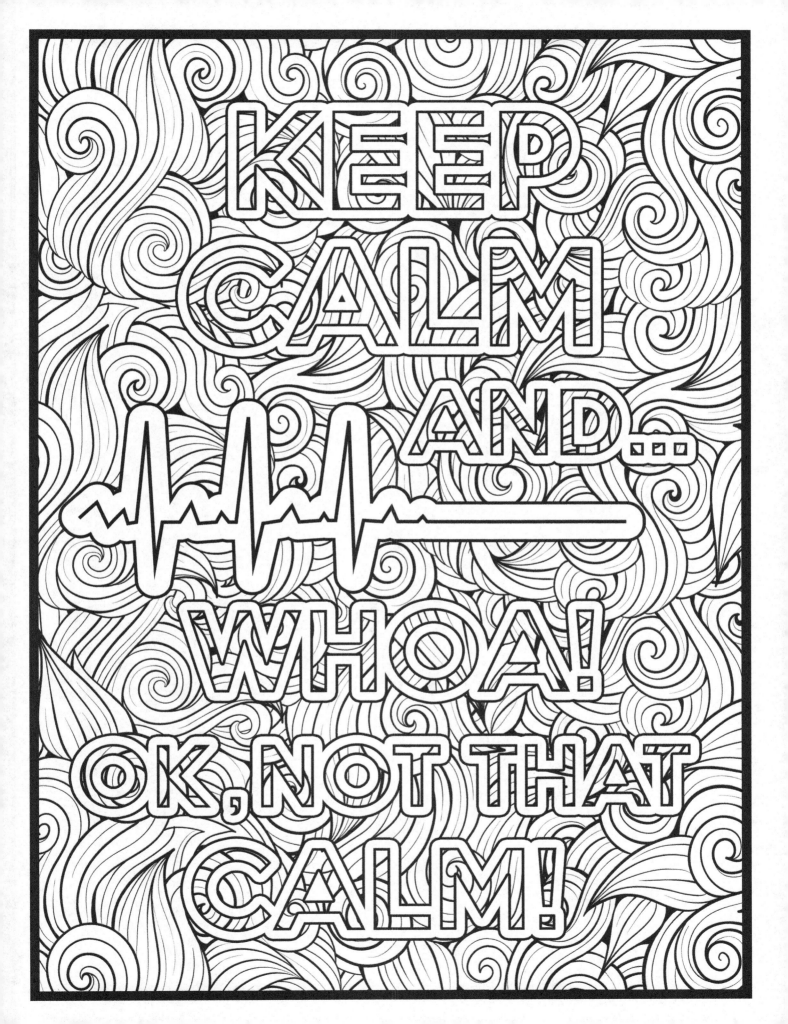

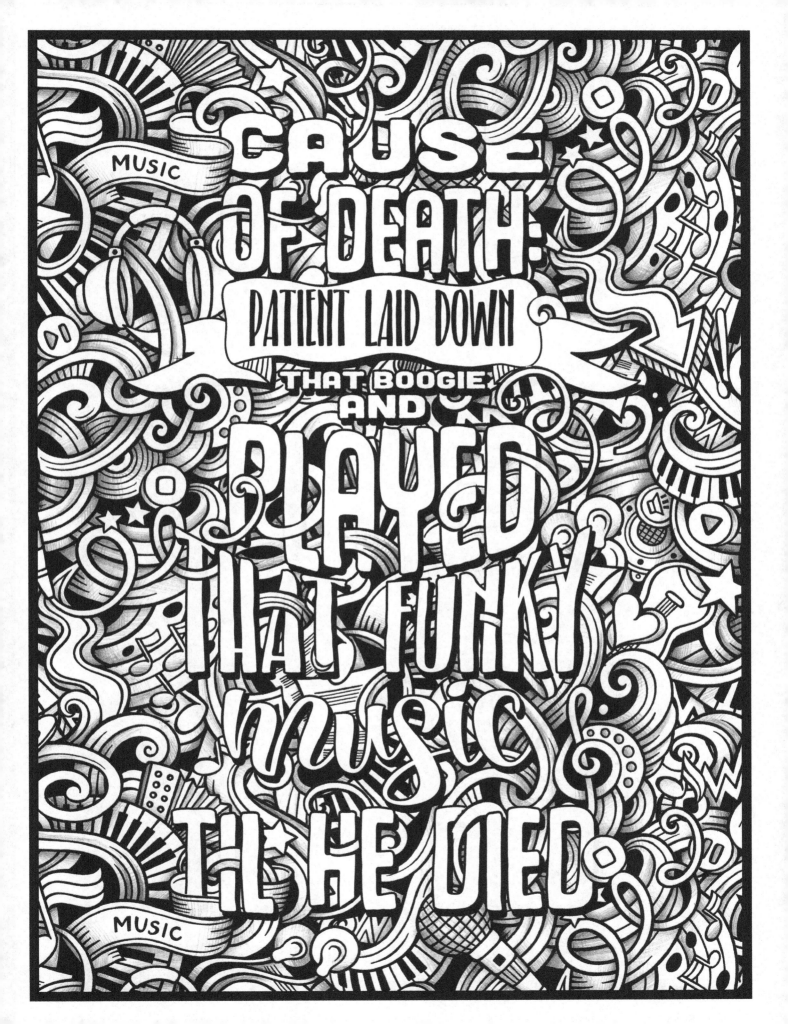

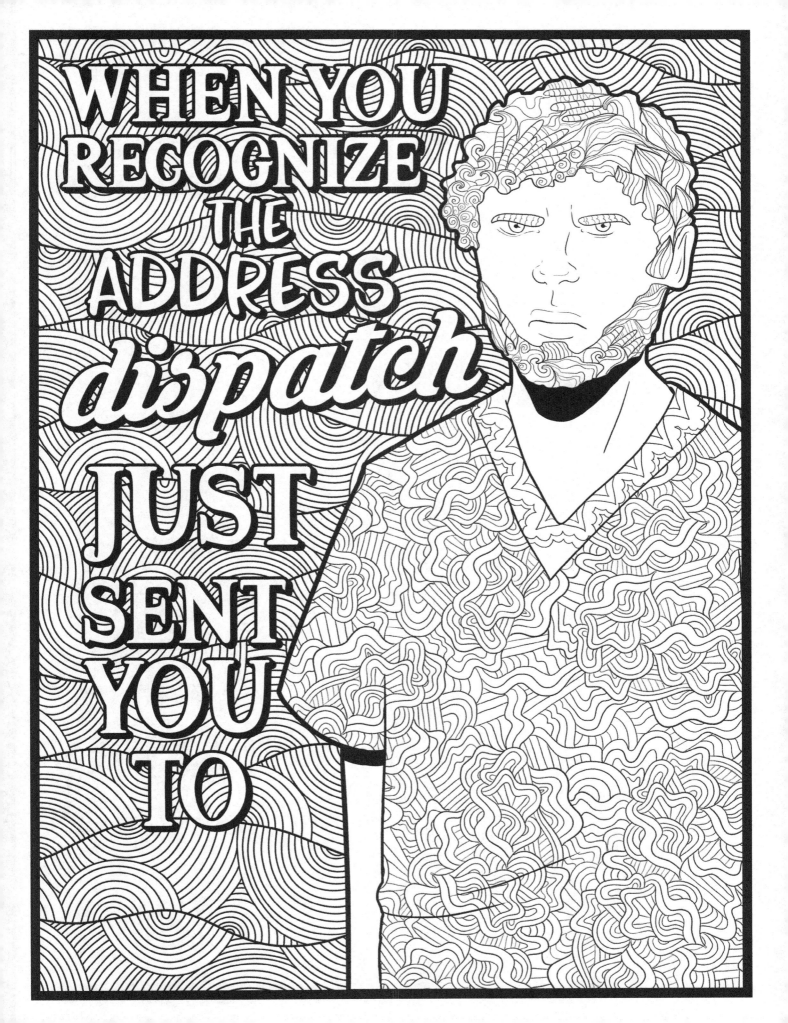

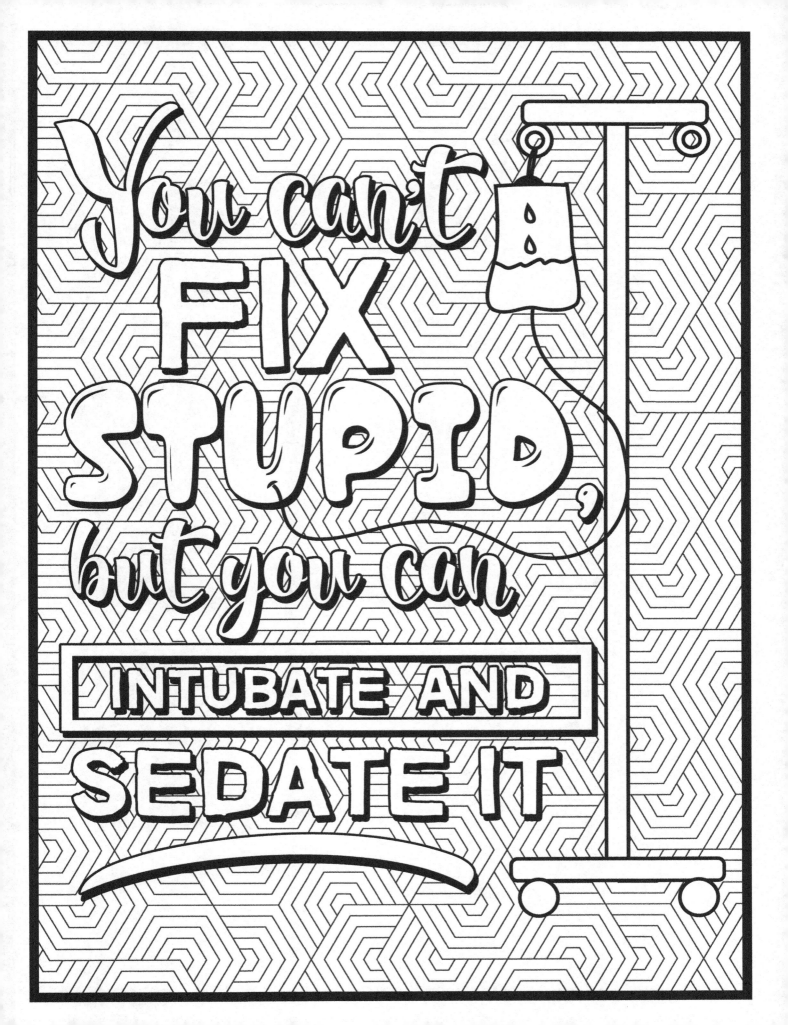

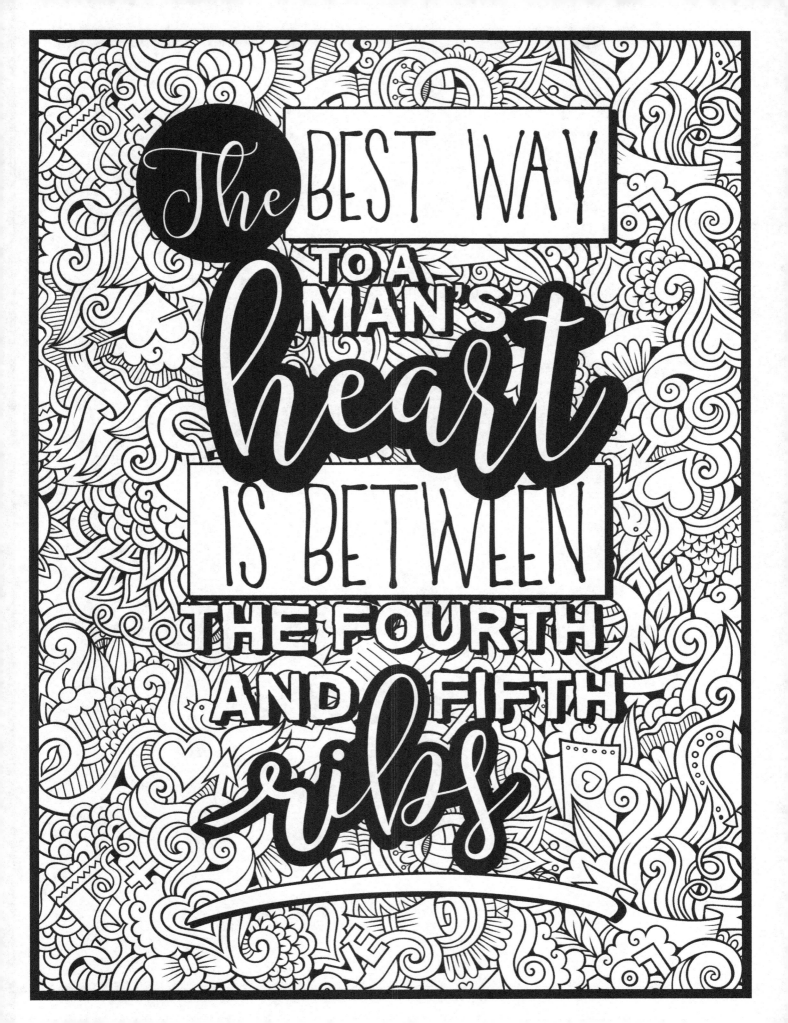

The BEST WAY TO A MAN'S heart IS BETWEEN THE FOURTH AND FIFTH ribs

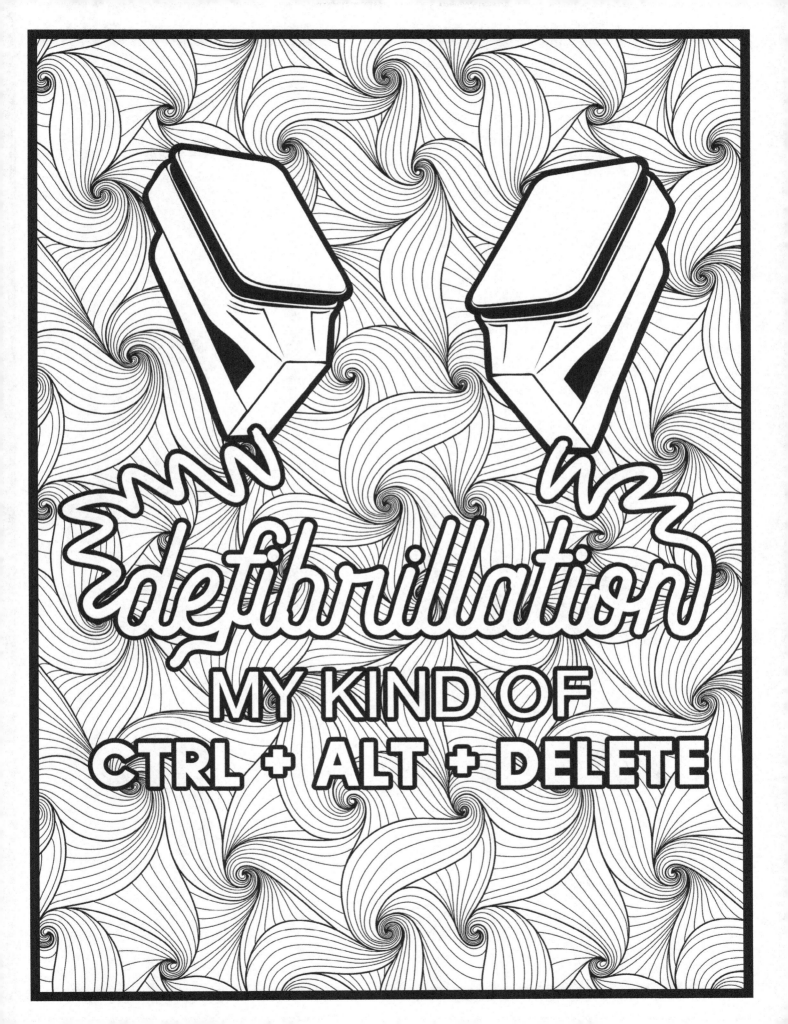

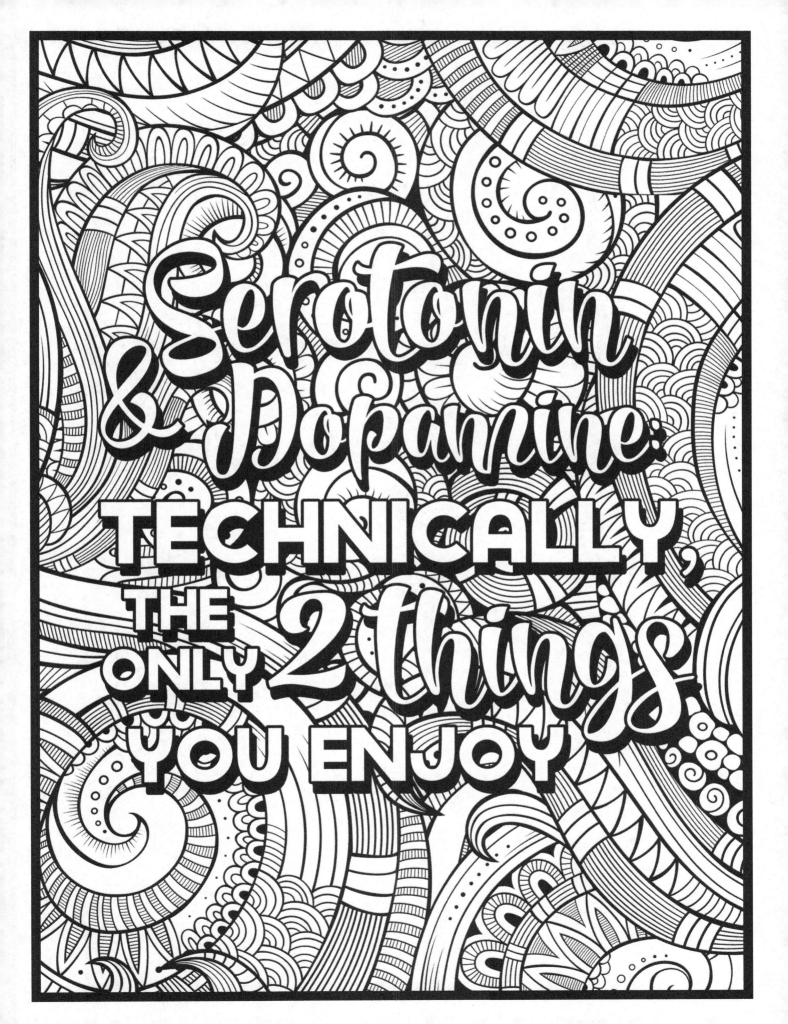

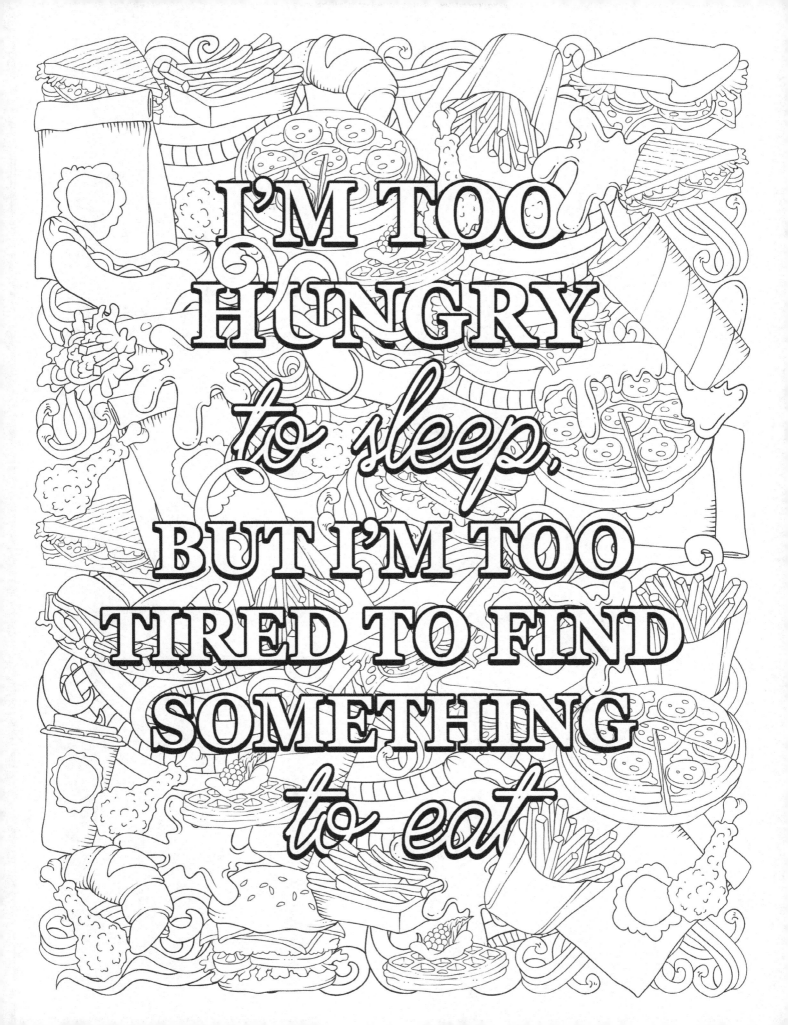

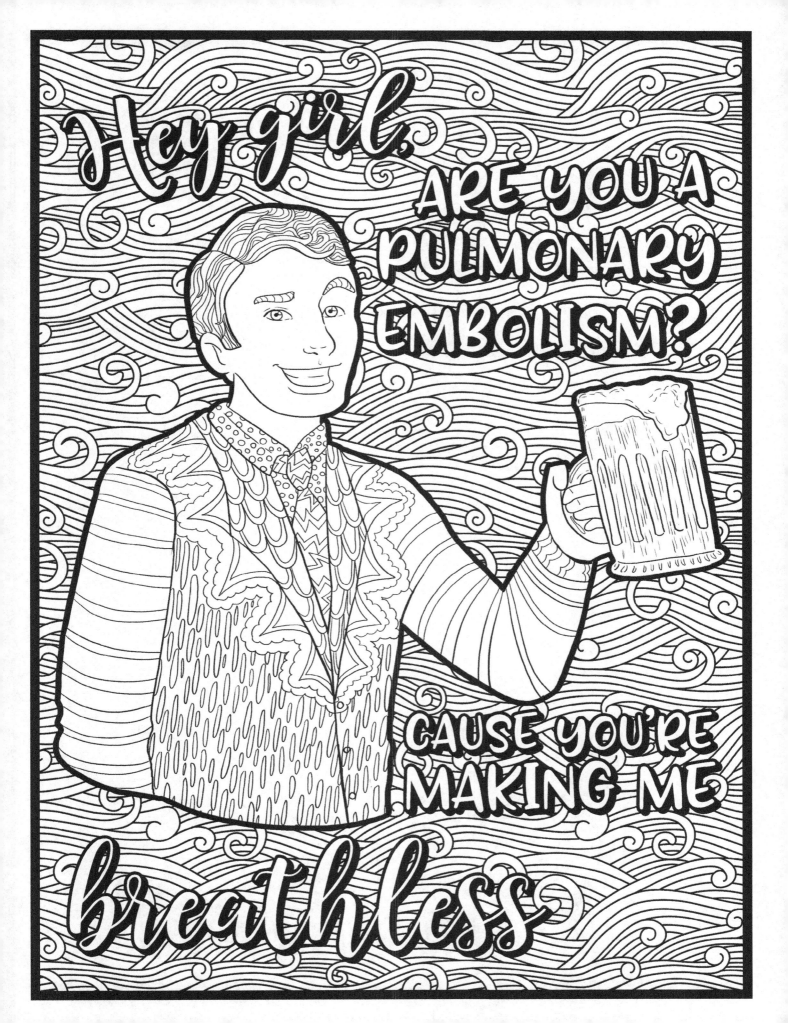

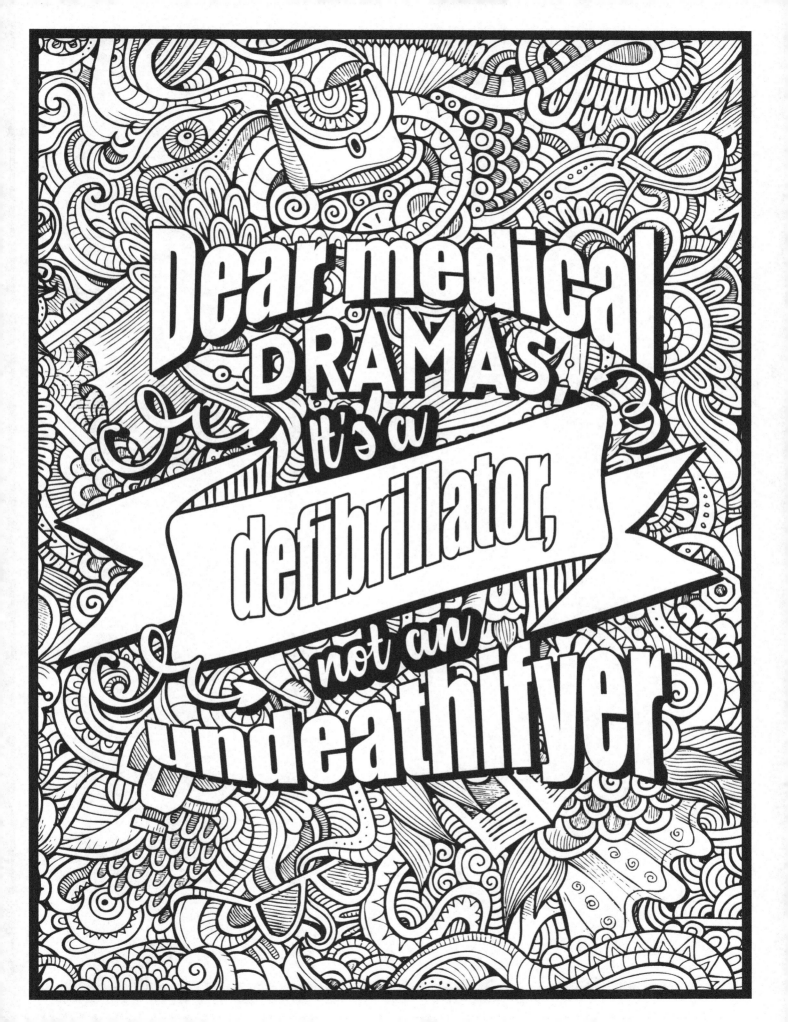

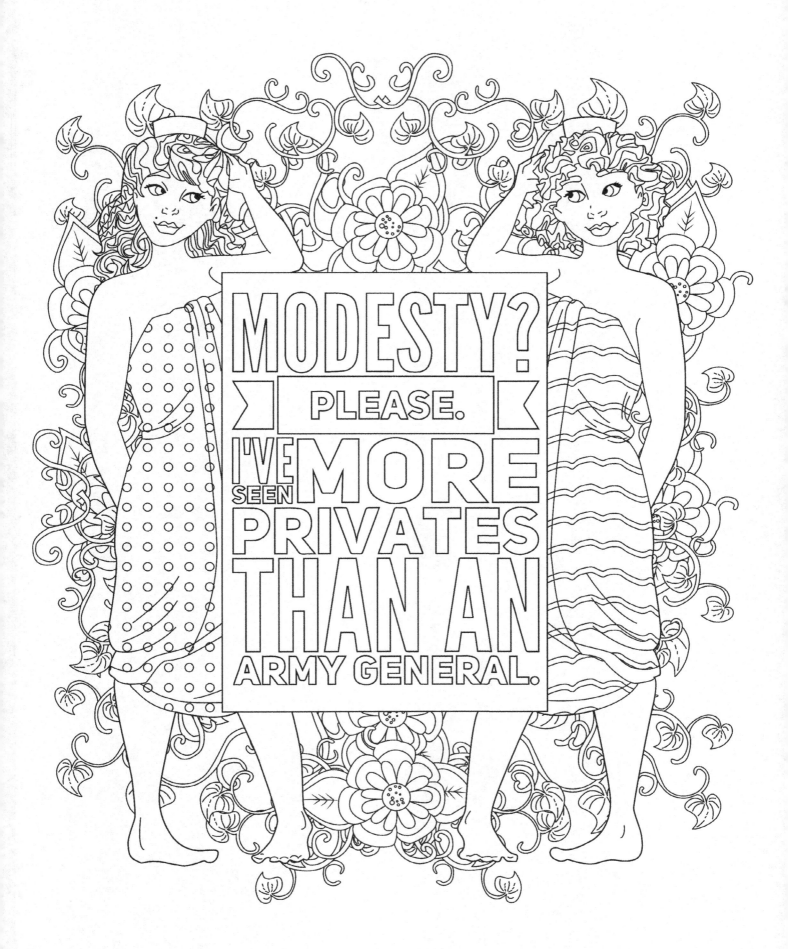

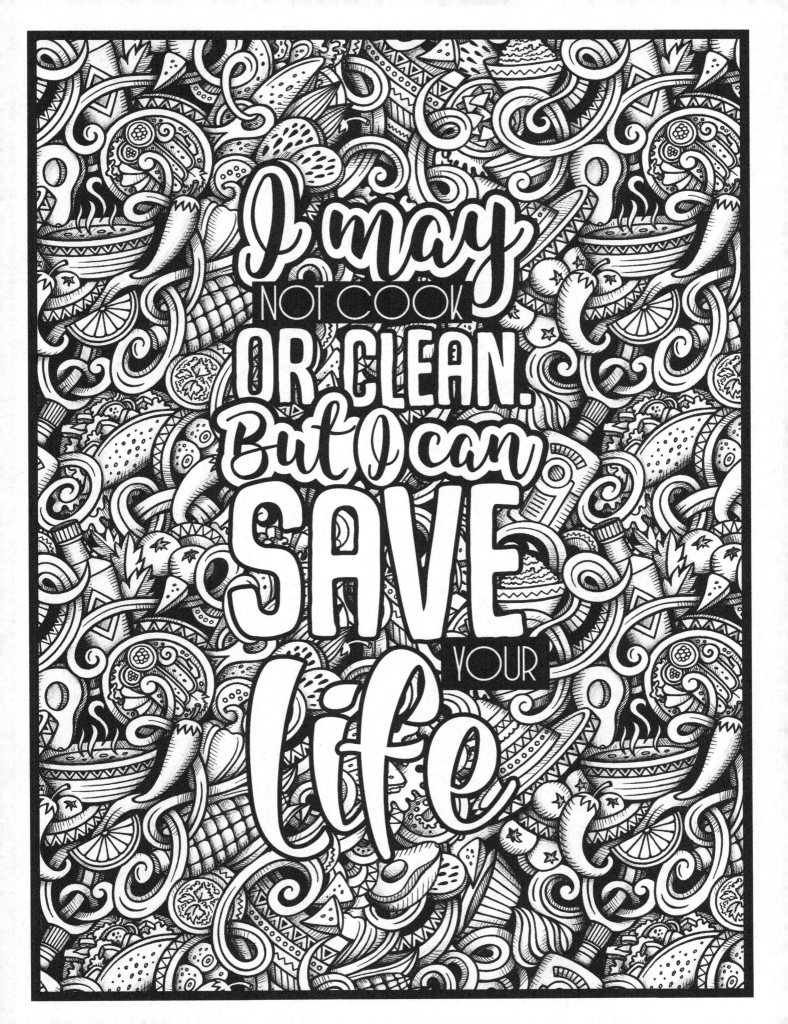

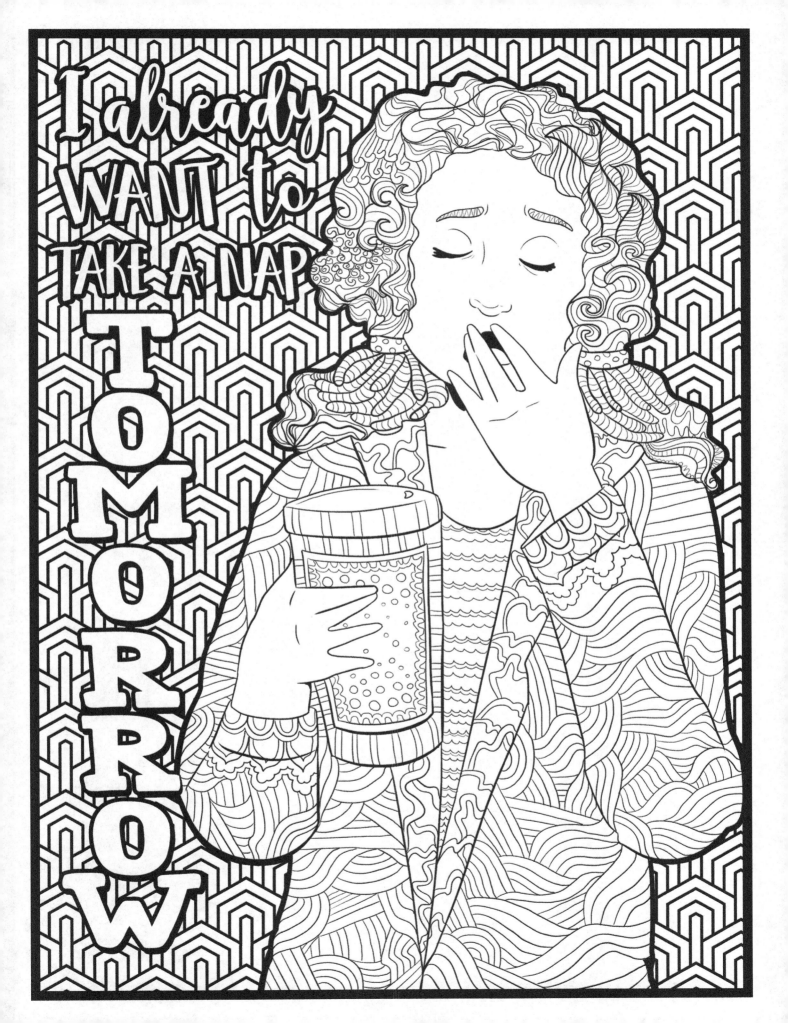

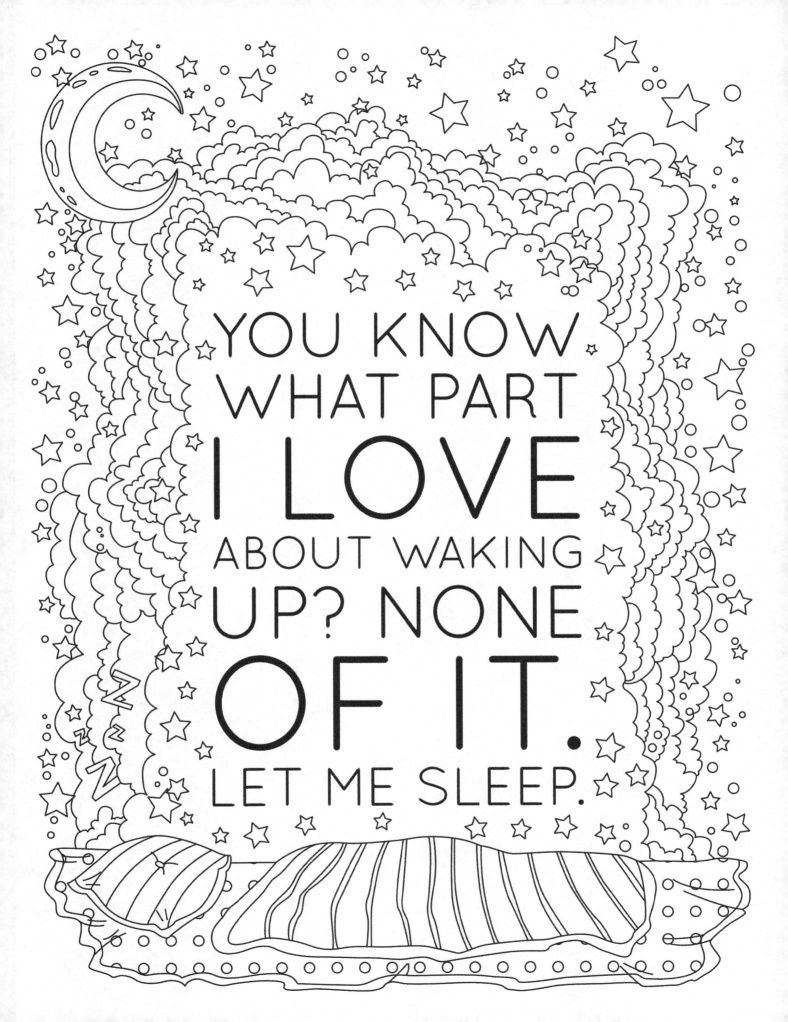

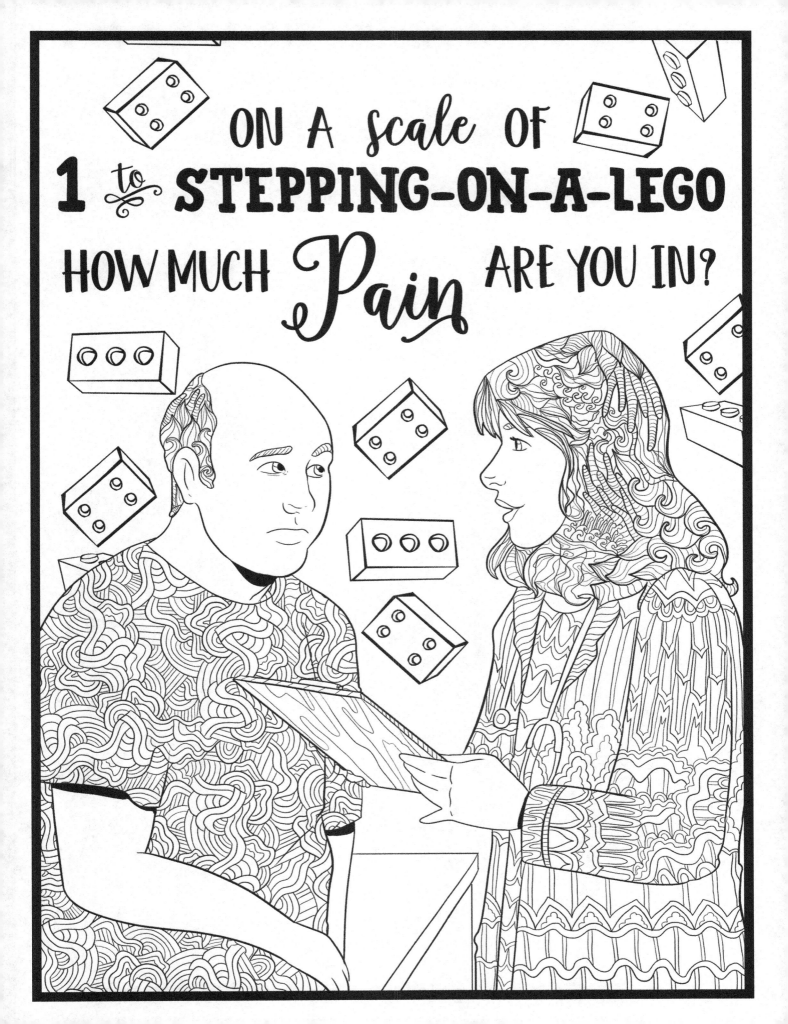

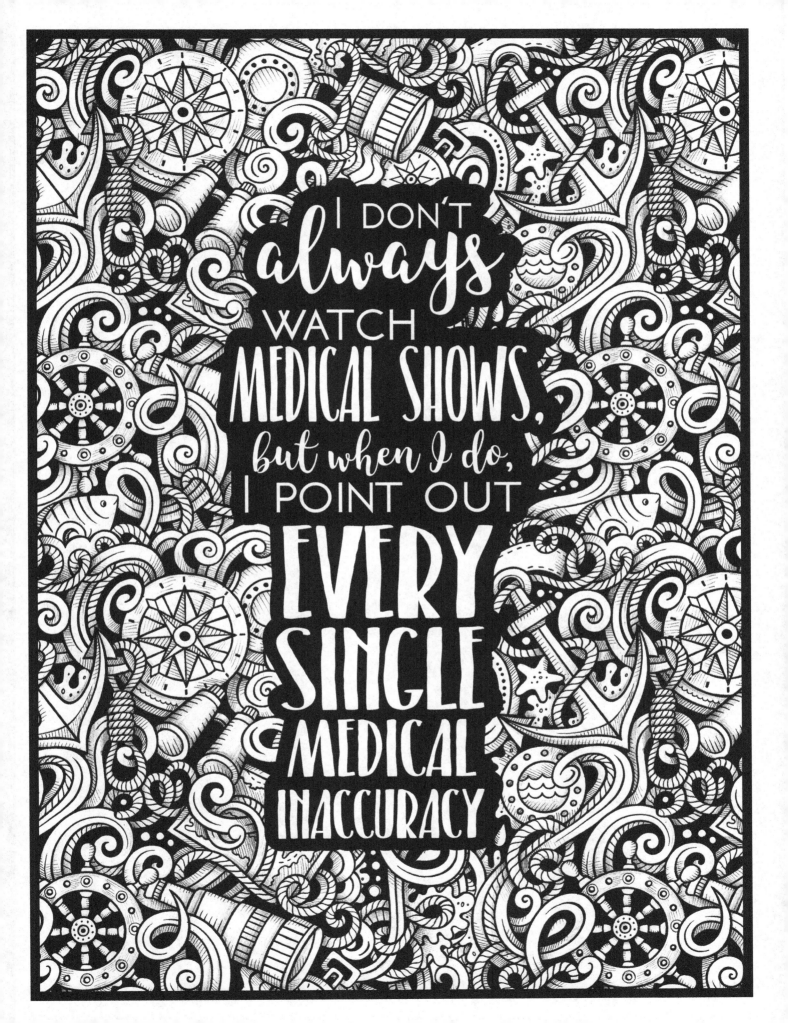

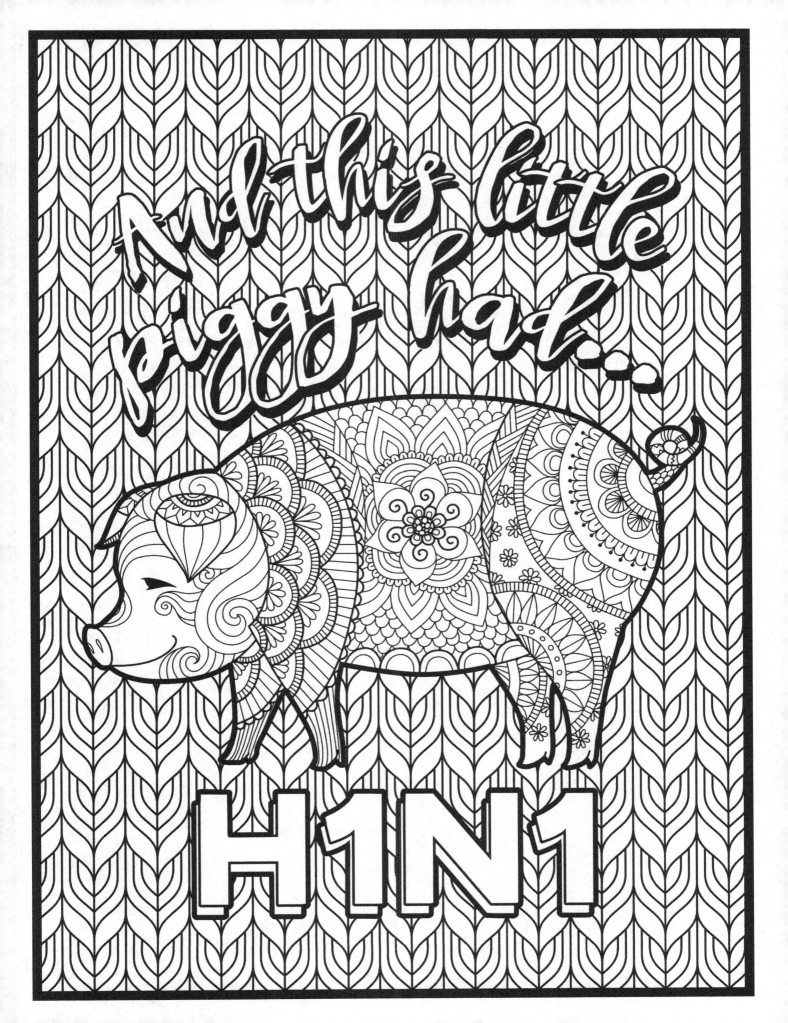

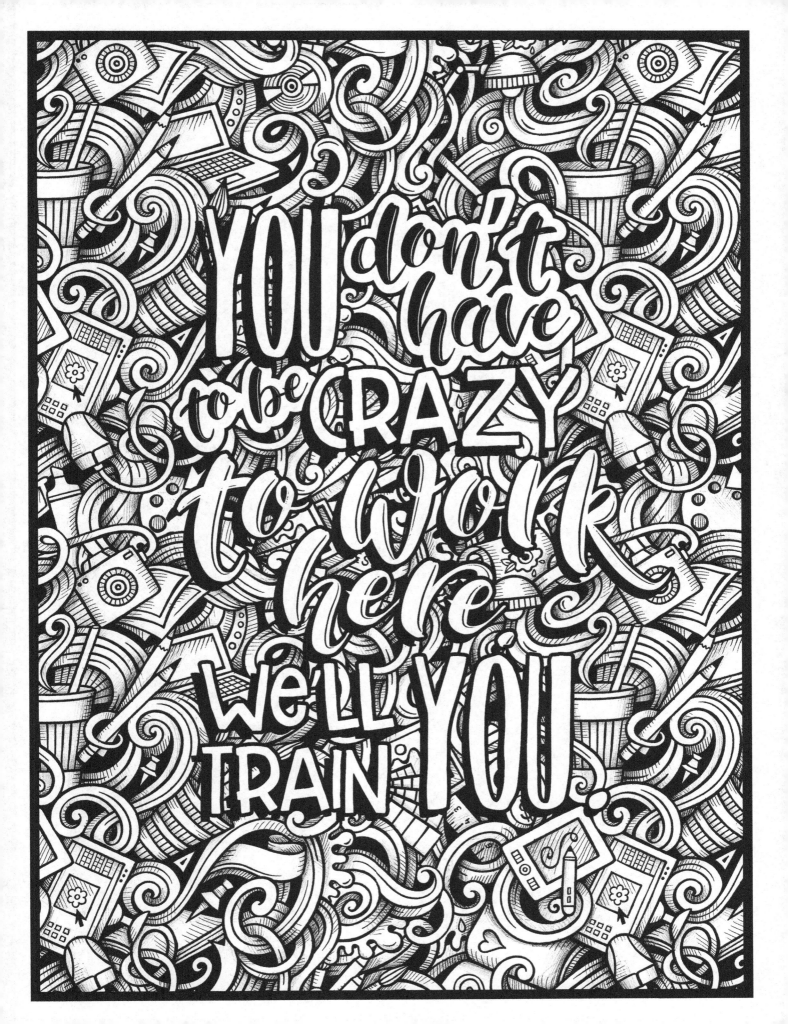

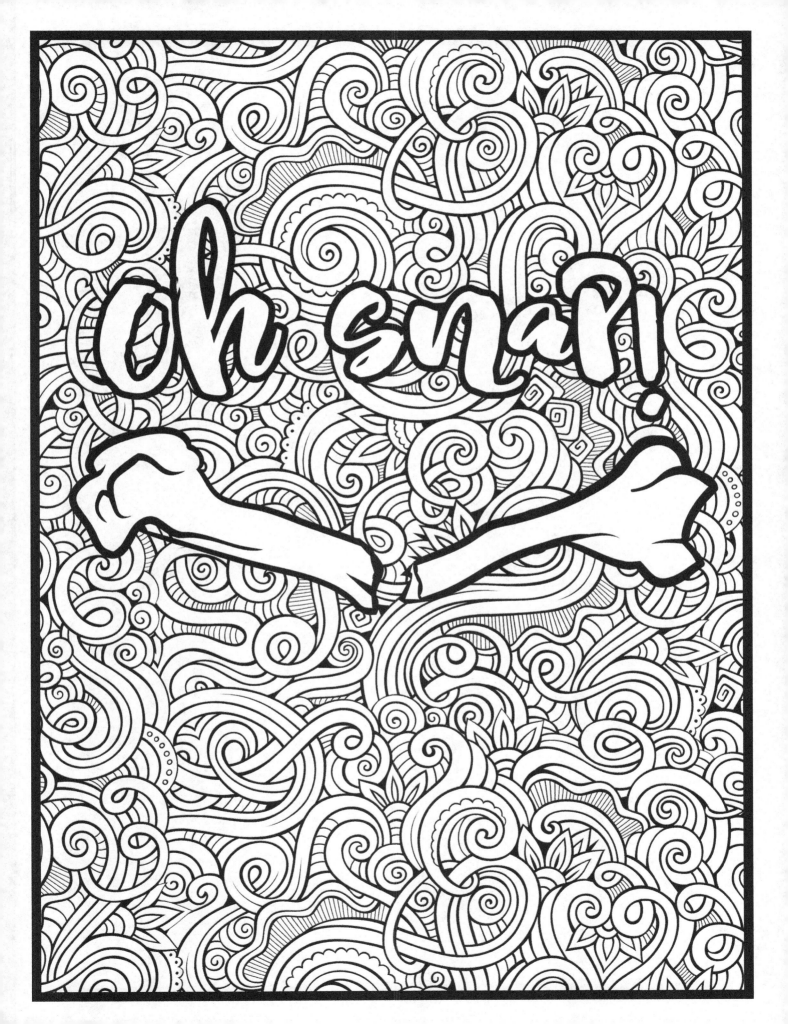

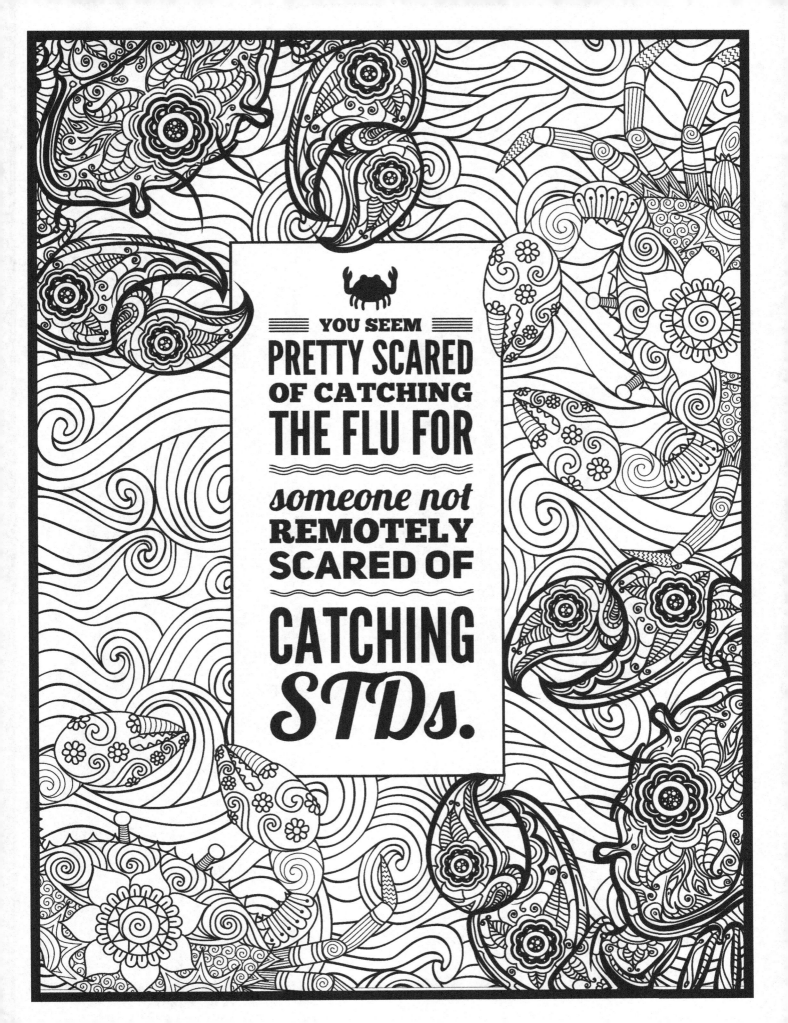

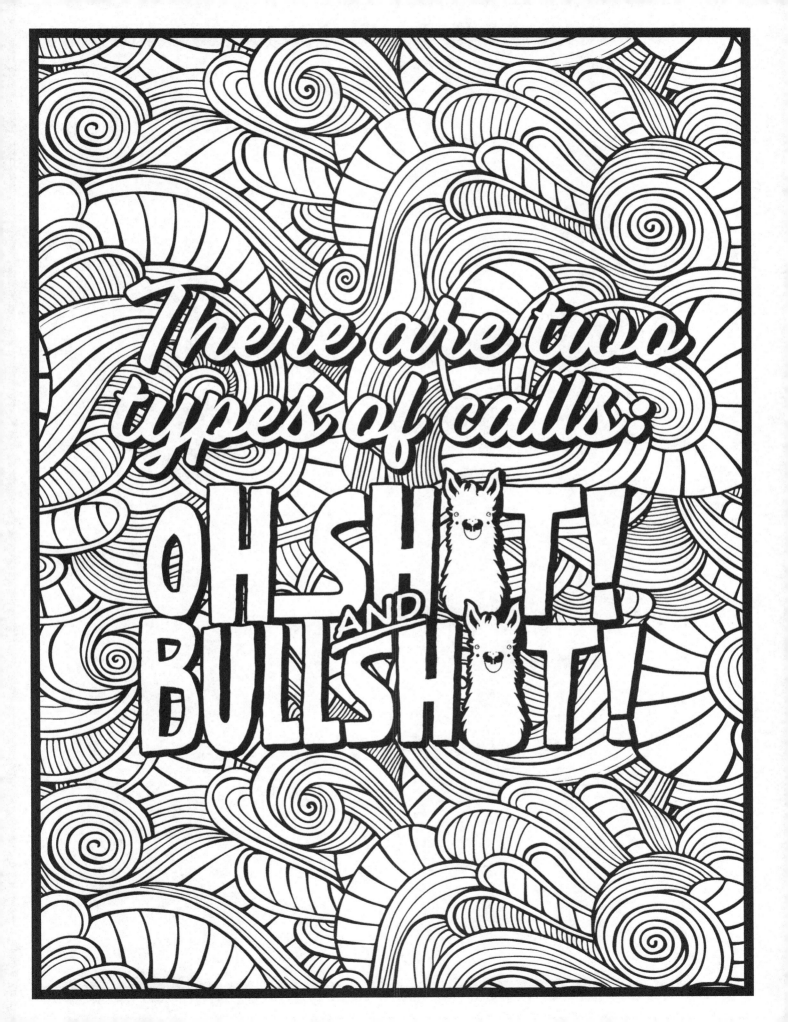

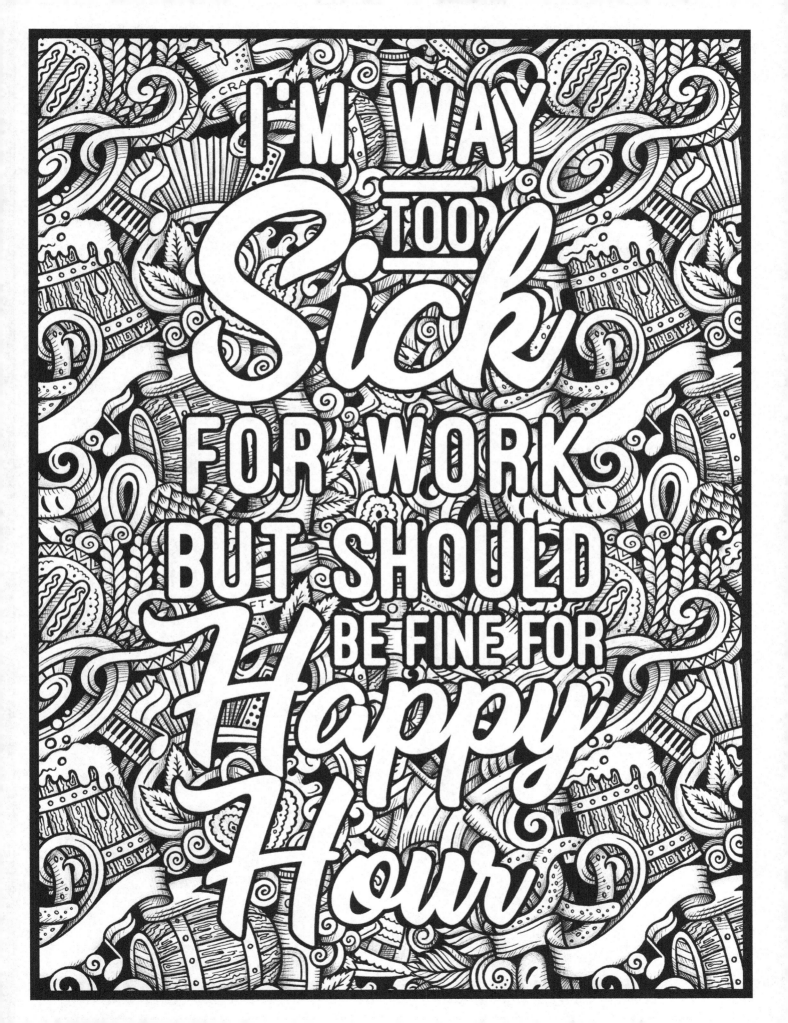

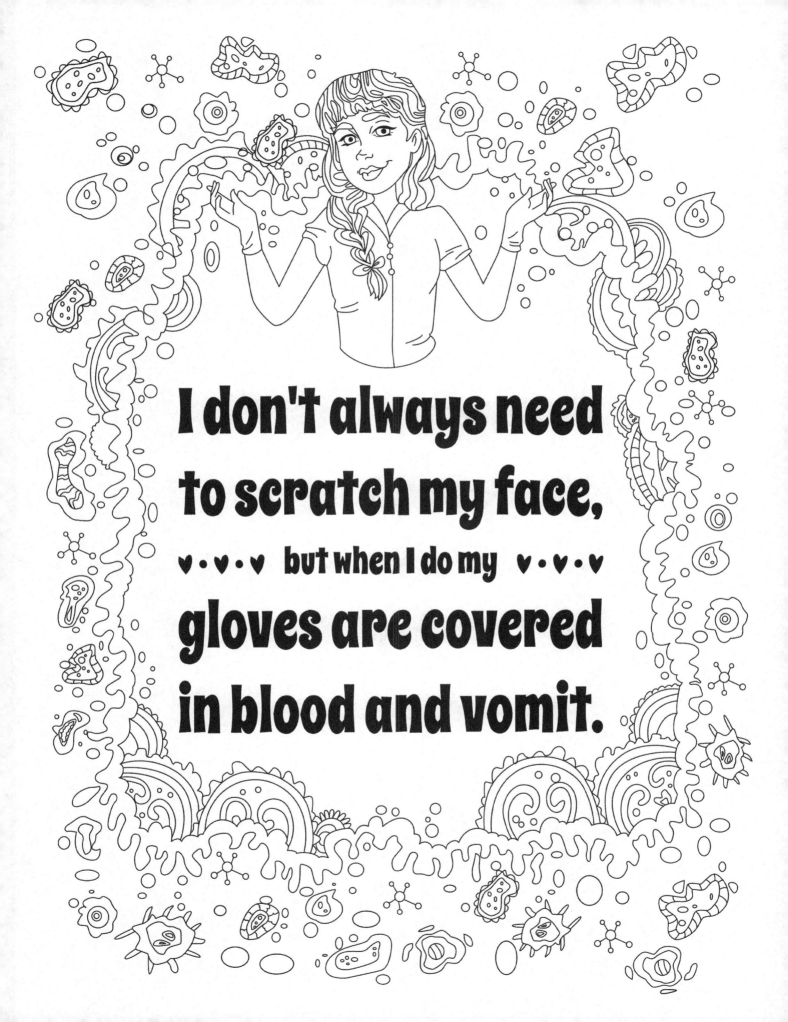

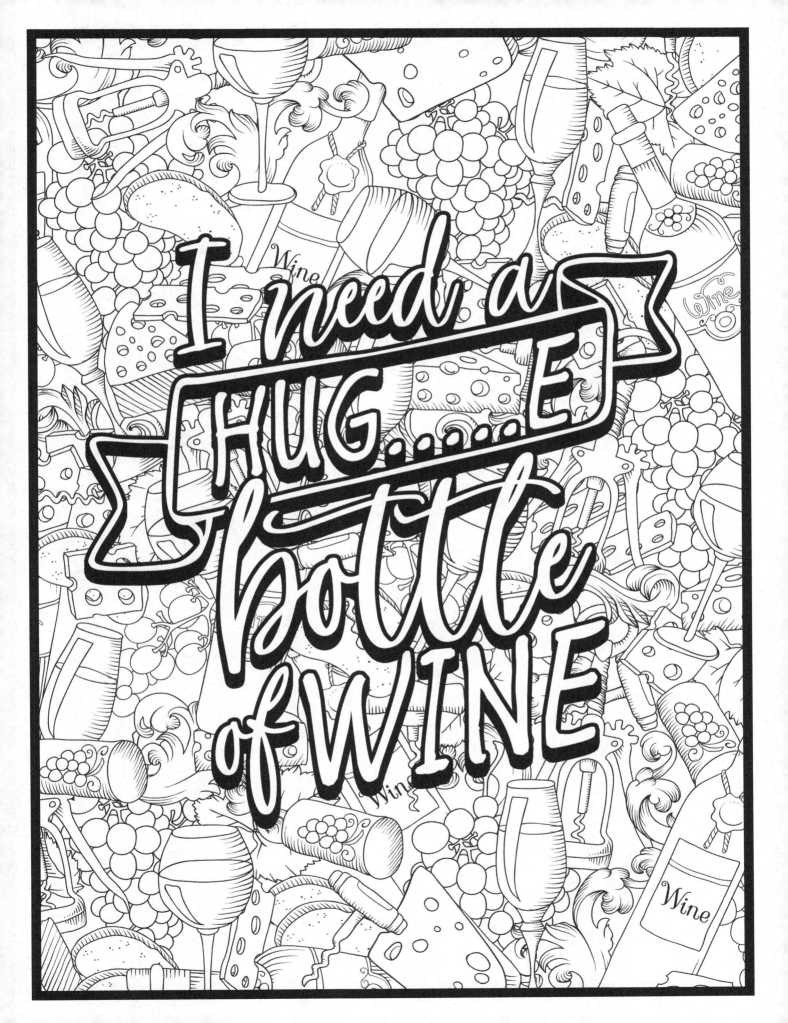

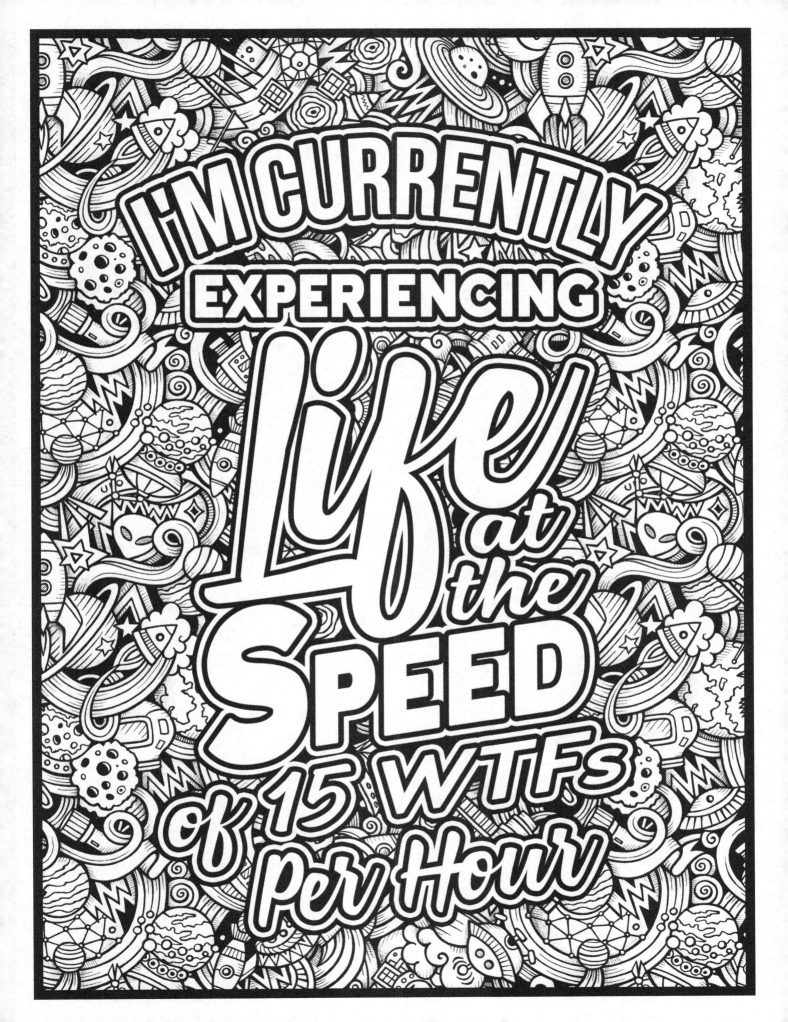

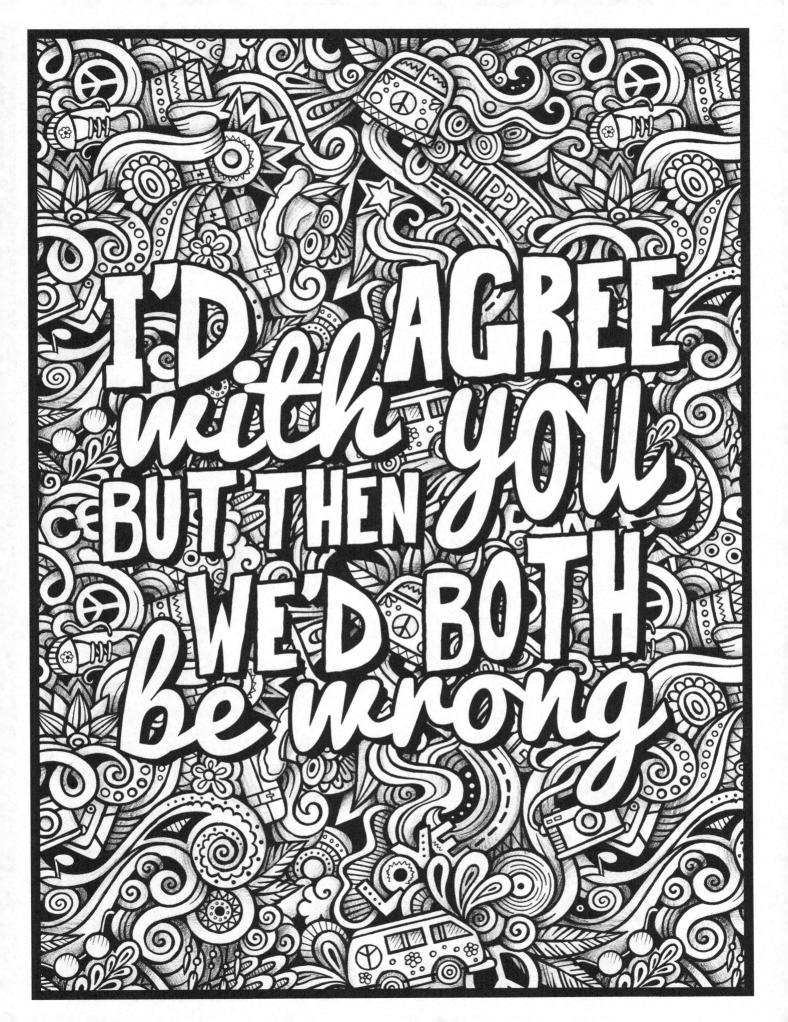

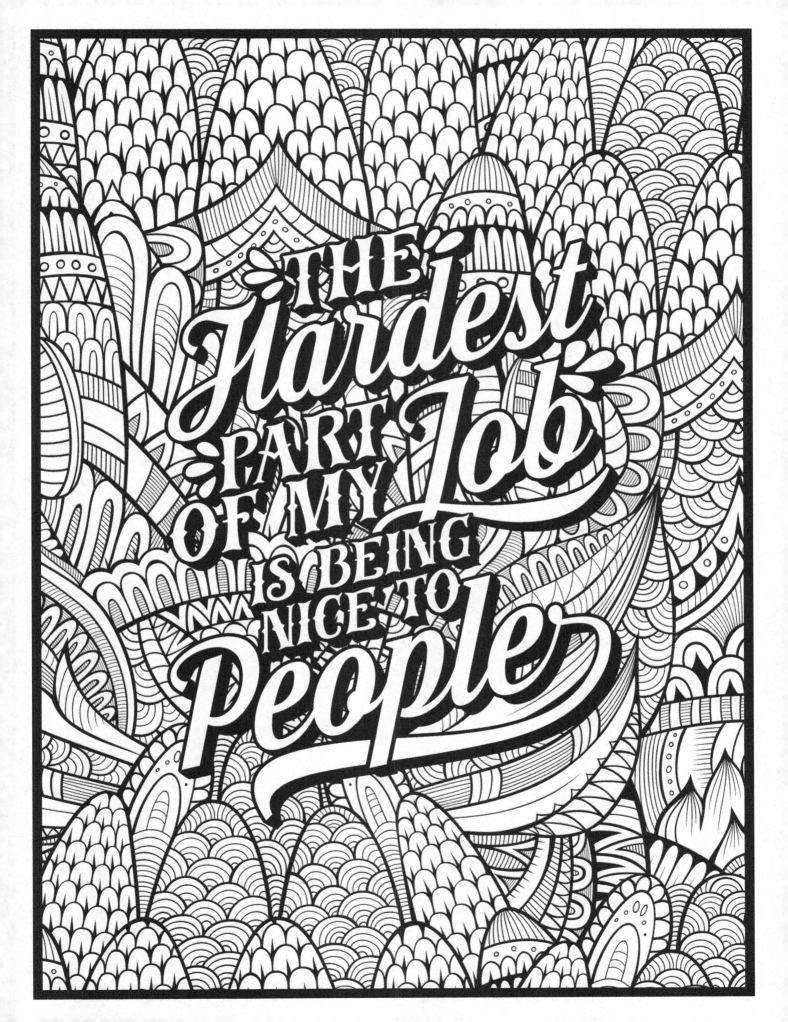

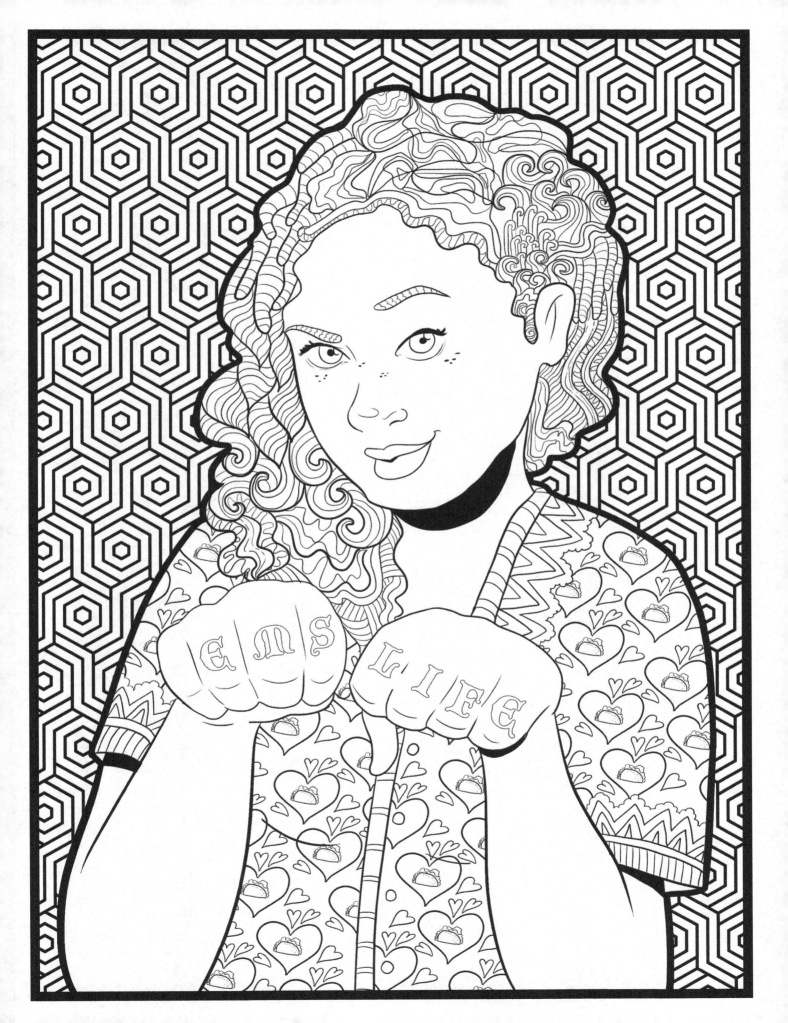

FREE PDF DOWNLOAD
OF THIS BOOK

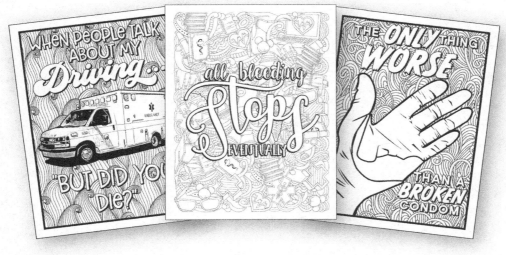

www.pbleu.com/ems

YOUR DOWNLOAD CODE: EMS373

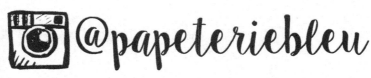 @papeteriebleu

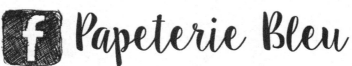 Papeterie Bleu

Want free goodies?
Email us at freebies@pbleu.com

@papeteriebleu

Papeterie Bleu

Shop our other books at
www.pbleu.com

Wholesale distribution through Ingram Content Group
www.ingramcontent.com/publishers/distribution/wholesale

For questions and customer service, email us at
support@pbleu.com

Made in the USA
Coppell, TX
26 August 2020

33907271R00063